# MEDICAL ERROR, ETHICS, and APOLOGY

Richard George Boudreau

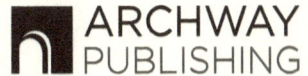

Copyright © 2020 Richard George Boudreau.

All rights reserved. No part of this book may be used or reproduced by any means, graphic, electronic, or mechanical, including photocopying, recording, taping or by any information storage retrieval system without the written permission of the author except in the case of brief quotations embodied in critical articles and reviews.

Archway Publishing books may be ordered through booksellers or by contacting:

Archway Publishing
1663 Liberty Drive
Bloomington, IN 47403
www.archwaypublishing.com
1 (888) 242-5904

Because of the dynamic nature of the Internet, any web addresses or links contained in this book may have changed since publication and may no longer be valid. The views expressed in this work are solely those of the author and do not necessarily reflect the views of the publisher, and the publisher hereby disclaims any responsibility for them.

Any people depicted in stock imagery provided by Getty Images are models, and such images are being used for illustrative purposes only.
Certain stock imagery © Getty Images.

ISBN: 978-1-4808-9061-9 (sc)
ISBN: 978-1-4808-9059-6 (hc)
ISBN: 978-1-4808-9060-2 (e)

Library of Congress Control Number: 2020908336

Print information available on the last page.

Archway Publishing rev. date: 6/23/2020

# CONTENTS

FOREWORD ..................................................................................ix
PREFACE....................................................................................xiii
INTRODUCTION..........................................................................xv

DEFINING MEDICAL ERROR ....................................................1
A Myriad of Definitions ..................................................................1
Medical Error—By the Numbers ....................................................6

A HISTORY OF MEDICINE, MEDICAL ERRORS, AND
LITIGATION ..................................................................................9
A Brief History of Medicine............................................................9
The Growing Cult of Secrecy: The Inability to Disclose ................ 13
To Err Is Human: Opening the Pandora's Box of Adverse Events..... 20
Legal Briefs: The Link between Medicine and the Law ................. 25

THE ETHICS OF PHYSICIAN DISCLOSURE ........................... 29
Obligation to Disclose: The Philosophers of Ancient Greece ........ 30
Hippocrates: Foggy Approach to Error Disclosure......................... 34
Ethical Models Today...................................................................... 38

## MEDICINE, APOLOGIES, AND LITIGATION: THE PRESENT ....42
Deny-and-Defend: A Culture of Secrecy ............................................ 43
Sorry, Not Sorry: Practitioners and Difficult Apologies ................ 54
The Impact of "Not Sorry" on Patients..............................................61
The Impact of "Not Sorry" on Physicians ......................................... 65

## ANATOMY OF AN APOLOGY................................................71
Definition ................................................................................................71
Benefits of Apologizing .........................................................................74
The Art of Apologizing......................................................................... 77
Types of Apologies ................................................................................ 79
A Reluctance to Own Up..................................................................... 84
Apology Laws—Do They Work? ........................................................ 88

## THE FAILURE OF MALPRACTICE LITIGATION ........................... 97

## ADR, MEDIATION, AND ARBITRATION ...................................... 111
Defining Alternative Dispute Resolution ........................................ 112
Mediation ..............................................................................................114
Arbitration ........................................................................................... 121
ADR in Light of Medical Error ........................................................ 125

## COMMUNICATION-AND-RESOLUTION PROGRAMS ........... 126
Rick Boothman, Defense Attorney .................................................. 128
Anatomy of a CRP—CANDOR........................................................ 132

## CAN DISCLOSURE WORK? CASE STUDIES ............................... 135
University of Michigan ...................................................................... 135

University of Illinois at Chicago ............................................................ 140
COPIC ....................................................................................................... 143
Additional Research ............................................................................... 144
Successes and Challenges ....................................................................... 145
Effectiveness and Rollout ....................................................................... 150
The Disclosure Process .......................................................................... 152
All Disclosure, All the Time ................................................................... 153

## APOLOGIZING AND LITIGATION ........................................... 155
What Wronged Patients Need ............................................................... 156
Steps of an Effective Apology ................................................................ 159
Empathy .................................................................................................. 165
Necessary Training ................................................................................. 166
Involving the Patient .............................................................................. 168
Sorry Works! To an Extent ..................................................................... 170
Implementing Enterprise Risk Management ..................................... 173

## DISCUSSION .................................................................................... 181
## REFERENCES .................................................................................. 185
## INDEX ................................................................................................ 203

# FOREWORD

Poor or unexpected medical outcomes have become a lightning rod for blame and litigation, especially if communication of essential information is lacking. In this age of advanced technology in the diagnosis and treatment of disease, what appear as medical errors are compounded by our dysfunctional and largely impersonal healthcare system. The latest pharmaceuticals and treatments developed for the multitude of genetic and epigenetic issues we face are too often sullied by the media, while ignoring inherent dangers and consequences (read as the frequently understated "black box warnings").

With the enormous explosion of technology comes an overwhelming amount of information and disinformation. With the erosion of the nuclear family and the present political divisiveness, there is loss of trust and conviction. Litigation has become a reflexive solution to our ills with its frustrations and siege mentality in which we find ourselves. This is especially true of the physician, who has the demoralizing task of working with an electronic health record that steals time from patient care, education conferences and even lunch. The corporate takeover of healthcare with the complicity of the health insurers and the laissez-faire attitude of our government concerns itself primarily with the bottom line.

Dr. Richard Boudreau is absolutely correct with his analysis of our failure of medical error disclosure: in the present "conspiracy of silence" with its "deny and defend" mantra that largely permeates our medical world, the path toward empathy must begin with the acknowledgement of a bad outcome. "I'm sorry" should not suggest guilt but must be timely and freely offered with the best information. Hospitals and personnel must have a mechanism to acknowledge a complication with follow through until all pertinent discussions are completed. Legal reform is needed, so litigation due to this conspiracy of silence and inordinate delays for justice can be overcome.

Dr. Boudreau explains so well the hazards and delays of litigation, the mechanics of mediation and arbitration and the no-fault approach offered by the COPIC Insurance Co. Corporations that mandate mediation and/or arbitration too frequently have an unfair advantage in winning cases (e.g., Kaiser, other HMOs, hospitals) as they have ready access to the best legal minds.

To coordinate the ideal program of forgiveness, a healthcare system must allow transparency with the mechanism for acknowledging the injured, cover their recovery and possibly compensate them (with a review board); no-fault insurance does not work as it is too readily gamed.  Physicians, especially overworked residents in training, may spend 10 minutes or less daily in direct patient care and too much mandatory documentation. Nurses are also engaged too long at the computer documenting charges and not enough time with the patient. Medical workers must be relieved of this repetitive and wasteful electronic burden. By allowing physicians and nurses the necessary time for a meaningful relationship with their patients, medical error should diminish and outcomes improve. The "wall of silence" must be replaced with better communication and easily accessible information that allows the patient to heal and have the confidence that healthcare should offer.

Dr. Boudreau has created a classic treatise with his book "Medical Error, Ethics & Apology." Hopefully, a future revision can highlight the subtitle, "It Is Always Safe to Say You're Sorry."

Jerome P. Helman, M.D.
Board Certified in Internal Medicine and Gastroenterology
Adjunct Assistant Professor in the Providence John Wayne Cancer Institute
jeromehelmanmd@gmail.com

# PREFACE

Deny-and-defend, as exemplified by the story of Beth Daley Ullem and the death of her newborn son from medical error, is a common way in which physicians and health-care organizations deal with the fallout from medical error. The problem, however, with the deny-and-defend stances is that failure to acknowledge a medical error to a patient or to apologize for it (with appropriate compensation) is likely to lead to a costly, ongoing lawsuit that neither patient nor physician can afford.

Today's ethicists and medical scholars agree that disclosure to patients and their families in the aftermath of an adverse medical event is required. The problem, however, is that defining what exactly medical error is can be difficult. Furthermore, the practice of medicine is inherently dangerous. And finally, the history of both medicine, and medicine and litigation, continues to ensure that physicians and hospitals are likely to keep mum in the face of an adverse medical event.

It shouldn't be that way, however. This book examines the concept of medical error / adverse medical events and how apologies and disclosure can help ultimately reduce litigation costs that could be inherent in such a situation. The book examines why litigation is an absolutely wrong way to deal with medical error and delves into the practice of apologizing. Other topics focused on include the culture of deny-and-defend, different methods of resolution other than litigation, and the effectiveness of communication-and-resolution programs. The ultimate focus of this book is that, while simply saying, "I'm sorry," is a good step when it comes to preventing litigation in the face of a medical mistake, that apology needs to be delivered correctly (through training) and should be part of a formal disclosure program for it to be effective.

# INTRODUCTION

When Beth Daley Ullem's newborn son, Michael, died from a medical error, she was understandably devastated. No one expects to go into a hospital to give birth only to come out of that experience without a baby to hold, love, or nurture. However, when her baby died, all Daley Ullem wanted to know was why it happened. She wanted an investigation into what went wrong and why the situation happened and an assurance from both the hospital and her doctors that actions would be taken to prevent the same errors from happening again to other families. A lawsuit was the last thing on her mind; her goal was simply to understand how "you're going to improve and protect families" (Smith, 2019).

Rather than getting a straightforward explanation and apology, however, Daley Ullem was stonewalled from getting any kind of information from the start, with an attitude she dubbed as "complete deny-and-defend." The hospital offered no investigation, no answers, no apology, no assurance of improvement, and no indication that the error wouldn't happen to another family. To make matters worse, Daley Ullem learned that the event was hidden from the hospital's quality department. "To me, that was going from error to insult," she commented.

Plus, this particular hospital in question didn't have an exactly stellar record when it came to similar events. As a former claims processor for a consulting firm, Daley Ullem was well aware of this institution's poor record of medical errors and costly claims. When her son died, Daley Ullem recognized the pattern of claims against the hospital as well as the conspiracy of silence surrounding the event.

After her son was buried, Daley Ullem tried to get to the bottom of what had happened to him, both because she wanted to know and because she hoped to prevent similar issues from happening to other families. The response she received, however, was less than exemplary; she was told "sometimes bad things happen." Beyond that, nothing more was said. Furthermore, insult was added to injury as the hospital continued sending bills to her for her $90,000 cesarean section. In short, Daley Ullem lost her child, she was never told why the incident happened, her attempts to get to the bottom of the situation were met with silence, and then the hospital decided it was a good idea to bill her for services. All this prompted her to make the difficult decision to sue the institution.

Suing the hospital also led to some interesting events—for one thing, the hospital actually went out of its way to destroy Daley Ullem's computer records and fetal monitoring strips (Smith, 2019). The good news for the bereaved mother was that she won the day and put the $4 million settlment into a fund to be used for projects and promotions related to a communication-and-resolution program (CRP).

In telling her story, Daley Ullem reiterated, several times, that the last thing she wanted to do was sue the hospital. All she wanted was answers and an apology. The hospital, however, didn't issue either of those, going out of its way to make life more difficult for her, the result being that she felt she had no choice but to take legal action in an effort to get some answers. In the aftermath of the suit and victory, she pointed out that patients aren't looking for perfection, but they do want a commitment to patient care and honest communication, especially in the aftermath of an adverse medical event. "I think people are remarkably forgiving if you say right away, 'here's what happened, here's what we're going to improve, and we're not going to hide from you.'"

While Daley Ullem's situation might seem somewhat extreme when it comes to the treatment of physicians or hospitals in the event of an adverse medical error, it's common for silence to be the response, along with a lack of accountability. Most health-care organizations tend to be opaque and nonforthcoming when it comes to admitting wrongdoing and apologizing for it when adverse events take place. This flies against ethical and moral obligations we have as human beings to each other when we have inadvertently wronged someone else.

The practice of medicine might seem to be, on the surface, one that is exotic and certainly one that can be dangerous and risky. Physicians and other health-care providers carry a great deal of responsibility when it comes to caring for patients and ensuring their continued good health. Yet, when it comes right down to it, health care is an industry, one that delivers services to meet the demand of patients. That service is offered for payment, whether that payment is "self-pay" or through a third-party payer. Yet when a mistake takes place in other industries, those who have made the mistake will apologize, explain what happened, and rectify it (through some kind of compensation mechanism, such as giving the customer his or her money back). If the business owner and employees are especially forthcoming, they'll also let the customer know that steps will be taken to ensure the mistake doesn't happen again. This is a necessity as a business, especially in this day and age of social media; they don't want to lose business because of an inadvertent mistake.

However, in the health-care universe, when an adverse event takes place, one that might affect the patient's quality of life or even lead to that patient's death, the patient and his or her family might end up in a position that is similar to Daley Ullem's. In other words, the patient or his or her family might face a wall of silence, the pretense that nothing happened and no one is to blame for it. The health-care establishment, and physicians working for it, might deny involvement with the error, while continuing with business as usual—the end result being little to no improvement, more mistakes being made, and bewildered patients or families. And as in the case of Daley Ullem, frustration with that attitude and philosophy tends to lead to litigation, meaning lawyers become involved, and the issue and pain are dragged out over time as the process moves from discovery to depositions to an eventual trial by jury. This is no way to run the health-care industry, and it doesn't have to be this way.

Certainly, when a health-care practitioner makes a mistake or error, the corrective measure often involves more than some kind of refund. The extent to which medical errors can maim or otherwise compromise the patient's quality of life is both grand and far-reaching; that disclosure is not always forthcoming speaks to a multitude of personal and legal troubles the responsible party wants to avoid. For this reason, most patients harmed by medical error actually never learn about that error ("Disclosure of Errors," 2019). Physicians tend to judge the importance of an error—and subsequent disclosure—based on whether it actually causes harm to the patient (Chamberlain, Koniarus, Wu, and Pawlik, 2012). If an error doesn't seem to create any harm, they might be thinking, there is no reason to acknowledge it happened.

Another reason for silence in response to an adverse medical event is that there are few, if any, systems in place that allow acknowlegdment of errors or allow those who have committed the errors to take responsibility for them. Instead, more often than not, the focus is on assigning blame for the mistake rather than on a sincere effort to find out what caused it and how to prevent that mistake from happening again.

The end result is what Daley Ullem faced: the deny-and-defend culture, one in which errors that are committed are swept under the rug and kept quiet. The potential repercussion of such errors, combined with the litigious society in which we live today, as well as the secrecy surrounding the health-care industry, means the admission of a mistake is going to be more the exception than the rule.

However, weighing the risk of potential litigation while at the same time respecting the patient's ethical right to know the truth presents a dichotomy that may be equally resolved with a simple two-word phrase: "I'm sorry." After all, when nonmedical businesses offer apologies for errors, most customers are forgiving.

As mentioned, however, the health-care industry is different. Certainly, reason dictates that a simple apology from a health-care provider to a patient for wrongdoing could help diffuse the problem and hopefully not bring the whole situation to the attention of a courtroom judge. And, to an extent, this is a good start. There is, however, in truth more to dealing with an adverse medical event than simply saying, "I'm sorry." The apology in and of itself needs to be more than an off-the-cuff effort. Furthermore, the apology needs to be issued in context with a disclosure, one in which the physician shares the truth of an adverse medical event with a patient or the patient's family. With these two factors in mind, the patient and family can recover from the event, the physician is able to get the issue off his or her chest, and the chances of litigation decrease exponentially.

The goal of this book is to focus on how apologies and disclosure programs can be effective, as well as why they are so necessary. The idea here is that a health-care organization needs to move from deny-and-defend to openness and honesty in an effort to help stave off costly litigation. This, in turn, will require an organizational change on the part of the health-care system and hospital.

As such, this book will focus on the following:

- the definition of medical error
- a history of medicine, litigation, and medical error
- the physician's ethical disclosure obligation to patients
- why the medical culture of secrecy makes apologies so difficult
- what patients truly want in the face of a medical error
- the challenges of litigation when it comes to seeking out the truth and obtaining information
- a solution: communication-and-resolution programs, mediation, and arbitration

- case studies outlining the success of various CRP and apology programs
- organizational change: the path to increasing disclosure and decreasing

The end result of this book is to

1) understand the physician's obligation to disclose error,
2) understand why it can be difficult for the medical establishment to admit wrongdoing, and
3) understand how disclosure and apologies in the face of adverse medical events can decrease litigation against physicians and medical establishments that have made mistakes.

The issue here isn't whether a physician will make a mistake. He or she will; physicians are, after all, human, and humans make mistakes. The issue is how the practitioner, and the organization for which he or she works, will handle the adverse event to ensure satisfaction on all sides, while reducing the need for litigation.

# DEFINING MEDICAL ERROR

### ◆ A Myriad of Definitions

MEDICINE IS A DANGEROUS BUSINESS, FOCUSED ON A delicate balance between life and death. There is both an art and science to practicing medicine, but even the best evidence-based practices can go awry. Certainly, mortality rates today are far less than they were even fifty years ago, thanks to advances in pharmaceutical research and technologies for treatment. But there is no such thing as a foolproof treatment.

For example, a fairly straightforward appendectomy is fraught with risk. Through such a procedure, a surgeon is physically cutting into a patient to remove an inflamed appendix. On the face of this, several things can go wrong. The wrong amount of anesthesia could be administered, causing brain damage or even death. The patient could be unknowingly allergic to the type of anesthesia, or even latex, creating further problems. A surgeon's hand could slip slightly, causing damage to surrounding organs. Despite the most hygienic practices, infection could seep into the wound, thus endangering the patient. The inflamed appendix could burst, causing additional problems. With all that could go wrong during this supposedly *simple* procedure, it's a miracle that the majority of patients are able to survive it.

The point here is not to scare anyone off from undergoing an appendectomy if needed. Rather, it's to prove that there is nothing simple about medicine and that things will go wrong. This can form the basis for our definition of medical error.

But there is more to the definition than the preceding. As we'll see, there are myriad ways in which this concept is perceived, which is one challenge when it comes to making an apology. Unless the concept of medical error is fully understood, it will be difficult to understand what to apologize for.

One common definition of medical error is either a failure of a planned action to be completed (in other words, an error of execution) or the use of a wrong plan or direction to achieve an aim or goal, which would represent an error of planning (Chamberlain, Koniarus, Wu, and Pawlik, 2012). A more clinically useful definition of medical error might be the following:

> A commission or an omission with potentially negative consequences for the patient that would have been judged wrong by skilled and knowledgeable peers at the time it occurred, independent of whether there were negative consequences. (Wu, Cavanaugh, McPhee, Lo, and Micco, 1997; p. 770)

Taking this further, medical error (or any kind of error, for that matter, outside of medicine) can either be active (commission) or passive (omission or inactive).

While the preceding provides a good basic overview of medical error or an adverse medical event, Grober and Bohnen (2005) aren't fans. These authors, who are practicing surgeons, point out that, at times, errors can be the result of outcomes influenced by actions outside of a health-care provider's control (Grober and Bohnen, 2005). The example these surgeons use is a patient with no known history of allergies suddenly experiencing an allergic drug reaction upon starting a new medication. Another example, getting back to our appendectomy, is a potential unexpected secondary issue that could reveal itself once the surgeon has opened the patient, such as an unknown infection, which could lead to further problems. "The outcome is unintended, yet not convincingly attributable to medical error," Grober and Bohnen note, adding that not all unintended outcomes can be attributed to medical error. These unintended outcomes aren't mistakes so much as they are unanticipated events, outside of a practitioner's control.

Given this, Grober and Bohnen suggest that medical error should be defined as "An act of omission or commission in planning or execution that contributes or could contribute to an unintended result."

Adding to the difficulty of pinpointing an exact definition of medical error, another layer is that such outcomes are rarely, if ever, singular events, especially depending on the complexity of treatment (Chamberlain, Koniarus, Wu, and Pawlik, 2012). If we take a step back from most mistakes, we find that this is true. If a mechanic makes a mistake in a car repair, it could be due to the fact that he or she is having an "off" day caused by lack of sleep or is dealing with a lot of extra cars on that particular day and, in his or her rush to get to them, might cut corners on all repairs. This might speak less to the propensity for error and more to the system that is supporting it. Perhaps the car repair shop should be more honest in telling customers when their repairs will be completed, so that the mechanic doesn't feel the need to rush to get through the processes.

In this case, auto repairs and patient repairs aren't too far off—they both operate within systems, and it's the strength of those systems that determines the preponderance of mistakes. Chamberlain et al. (2012) support this point, saying that medical procedures aren't performed in a vacuum—they typically involve a variety of decision processes and actions which could, in turn, be associated with problems or errors that might require attention. Focusing on our appendectomy mentioned earlier, it could be that the hospital or ambulatory surgery center is scheduling too many procedures in a given day. Or, perhaps, immediately previous to the appendectomy, the surgeon was faced with a life-or-death surgery that took a great deal of his or her energy or concentration, making him or her tired, irritable, and less focused on the fairly *simple* appendectomy to follow. Or if the anethesiologist is at fault, perhaps it was because she or he failed to ask the right questions of the patient or the patient's family before the surgery or didn't phrase the questions in the right way so the patient would understand how to answer. The end result could be an allergic reaction to the anesthesia. It's likely that these—and other—mistakes happen more often than not, but the majority of patients and their families are unaware of their occurrence. Generally, if the errors don't result in lasting harm to the patient, the slip-ups aren't disclosed.

Medical error can also be catagorized as a breach of a physician's duties. This breach can take many forms, as follows (Kass and Rose, 2016):

- misdiagnosis
- errors in choice or execution of procedures
- improper administration of medications
- failure to follow up appropriately with a patient
- failure to obtain adequate informed consent

Adding more complexity to the mix, an adverse event can be defined as an injury or other event that takes place by the treatment process, as opposed to the patient's underlying disease or injury (Helo and Moulton, 2017). This is in direct contrast to a complication, which is defined as "an unfavorable consequence of the patient's disease process" (Helo and Moulton, 2017).

As such, any one of the preceding could fall into the category of "medical error," which makes defending it or apologizing for it that much more difficult.

Physicians aren't the only ones who struggle with what, exactly, constitutes medical error or an adverse event. A study analyzing Canadian nurses working in long-term care reported that respondants had different definitions of what constituted harm through medical error; perhaps unsurprisingly, that perception affected whether the error was reported (Sorrell, 2017). See also Wagner, Damianakis, Pho, and Tourangeau, 2013.

Additionally, the Institute of Medicine, in its landmark report *To Err Is Human* (which I will cover in more detail later on), indicated that medical error and adverse events consist of a huge category that might include adverse drug events, improper transfusions, surgical injuries and wrong-site surgeries, suicides, restraint-related injuries, falls, burns, pressure ulcers, and mistaken patient identities. Trying to decipher which of these errors should be disclosed and even which of these events are actually errors can be difficult.

### ◆ Medical Error—By the Numbers

Because introducing an exact definition of medical error is difficult, getting a handle on the metrics connected with adverse events is also hard. In one study, it was estimated that only about 6 percent of doctors are responsible for approximately 60 percent of all malpractice payments; perhaps unsurprisingly, surgery errors tend to top that list (Anderson, 2017).

Another account indicated that as many as 98,000 patients die each year in the United States as a direct result of medical errors (Berlinger, 2008; see also Kohn, Corrigan, and Donaldson, 2000). From a financial point of view, another piece of research pointed out that preventable medical errors (in other words, those that could be avoided due to more effective systems control) cost the United States anywhere from $17 billion to $29 billion in health-care costs, lost income, and other expenses (Berlinger, 2008; see also Kohn, Corrigan, and Donaldson, 2000).

Some years ago, Makary and Daniel (2016) reported that medical error was the third-leading cause of death in the United States, a story that was carried throughout much of the mainstram media. The study, which appeared in the *British Medical Journal*, indicated that more than 250,000 deaths per year could be attributed solely to medical error (Makary and Daniel, 2016). In their study, the researchers took a look at four separate studies that analyzed the medical death rate data from 2000 to 2008. Then, using hospital admission rates from 2012, the researchers extrapolated that, based on a total of more than 35 million hospitalizations, more than 250,000 deaths stemmed from medical error—that makes up 9.5 percent of all deaths each year in the United States.

Gorski (2016) debunked these figures, pointing out that, for one thing, the *BMJ* piece is less a "study" and more an op-ed, given that it's an extrapolation of many pooled studies, with extrapolations based on smaller numbers. Furthermore, he went on to say that, given the definition the authors used in their piece, figures were inflated. Even as he counteracted the research and writings of Makary and Daniel, Gorski acknowleldged that, when it comes to medical errors, "we should do better" but won't do better by spreading myths or inflating figures.

The takeaways are the following:

1) One large problem when it comes to apologizing for medical errors (or putting an apology program in place for doing so) is that pinning down an actual definition of "medical error" is very difficult. Basically, if a patient comes to harm through an allergic reaction the physician didn't know the patient had, is this the physician's fault? Furthermore, if the error was the result of a system-wide breakdown in communication and action, who, in actuality, is at fault? And finally, should an error be disclosed, even if it was outside of the physician's purview?

2) The number of patients actually affected by medical error is also difficult to pin down. Depending on what definition is used for adverse events or medical error, the reality is we really don't know how many patients suffer from the results of medical mistakes. Because of this, it can be difficult to know what, exactly, to apologize for.

The idea here is not for practitioners to apologize for every little thing that goes wrong with a patient. Rather, it is to understand that, when mistakes do happen that could affect a patient's health, the deny-and-defend culture is not a way to prevent litigation. As such, a physician's desire to disclose an error will be based on 1) whether an event actually constitutes and error and 2) the degree of harm that takes place as a result.

But how did we get to the point in which physicians are unwilling to acknowledge any kind of wrongdoing? What will be helpful right now is to discuss a brief history of medicine and medical error and determine, from that history, why it has become so difficult for physicians to apologize for errors, leading to a culture in which lawsuits are not just the normal response for an adverse event but are expected.

As a note, before moving forward, I will frequently interchange the concepts of "medical error" with "adverse medical event" or even medical mistakes. All these lead to the focus of this book, which is an act of commission or omission that causes harm to patients.

# A HISTORY OF MEDICINE, MEDICAL ERRORS, AND LITIGATION

OUTSIDE OF TRYING TO PIN DOWN AN EXACT DEFINITION of medical error, understanding how we got here in the first place is helpful. The truth is disclosure has been a tricky business from as far back as prehistoric times. As such, understanding the history of both medicine and medical errors can be helpful in pinpointing the reluctance, today, of acknowledging wrongdoing.

### ◆ A Brief History of Medicine

**The First Humans**

It should probably come as no surprise that the practice of medicine as we know it today was vastly different in prehistoric times. When our ancestors were living off the land and more exposed than their current-day descendants to all kinds of disease and accidents, folk medicine and herbal remedies were predominant ways in which diseases were dealt with (Guthrie, Underwood, Richardson, Rhodes, and Thomson, 2019). A lack of understanding as to bodily functions ensured that magic and religion also played a large role in early human society's medical care; in many cases, it wasn't uncommon for early priests or rabbis to take care of physical ailments as well. But given the overall lack of sophistication of medical treatment at the time, if a person died from an accident or mistake, it might, more often than not, be attributed to some outside source (a higher power, such as God or gods) than the man (or woman) treating the individual.

### *Hammurabi—The First Legal Scholar*

The first mention of laws relating to the practice of medicine can be found in the Code of Hammurabi. I will be mentioning Hammurabi a great deal in this section because this eighteenth-century BCE Babylonian king's code arguably represents the first codified law that supports the basis of our legal decisions and information today. The code outlined the legal issues and decisions of ancient Mesopotamia, with a focus on criminal and civil matters. From a medical perspective, the code also offered a great deal of information, such as rates for general surgery and setting factors (for broken limbs), fees set according to a patient's ability to pay, the obligation of owners to pay for health care for their slaves, and objective outcome measurement standards to ensure quality of care for patients (Guthrie, Underwood, Richardson, Rhodes, and Thomson, 2019; see also Spiegel, 1997). Also, with a nod to universal health care, the code indicated that all the population was entitled to health care, no matter the social status, while also outlining credentialing procedures for health-care practitioners, which, at the time, included priests, veterinarians, barbers (who doubled as surgeons), and others (Spiegel, 1997).

The Hammurabi Code could be considered the first evidence of managed medical care in history, but it didn't really focus on whether health-care providers needed to apologize or whether they were necessarily required to disclose errors. The code did, however, indicate no margin for error; said Spiegel, "Health care providers had to be flawless or lucky," or otherwise suffer from various consequences, ranging from monetary fines to the rather overkill impalement on a stake. Deny-and-defend, which I mentioned at the outset of this book, and which I'll discuss later on, could likely have gotten its start in ancient Mesopotania, given the severe hazards for health-care providers who didn't do right by their patients.

### *Medicine Comes of Age*

As time went on, medical practices and their successes varied, depending on continent, culture, and technology. For example, traditional medicine in India included Vedic medicine (involving magic and charms), while health care in China focused on yin and yang balances (Guthrie, Underwood, Richardson, Rhodes, and Thomson, 2019). Yet once again, the practice of medicine had its roots more in the spiritual, rather than the physical; if something went wrong, it wasn't attributed to the practitioner but rather to high powers outside that practitioner's control.

The preceding focused on Eastern religions. The roots of Western medicine can be found in early Greece, which inherited much of its knowledge, in turn, from Babylonia—Hammurabi—and Egypt.

### Western Medicine and Hippocrates

The birth of Western medicine can be traced back to the Hammurabi Code, as well as ancient Egyptian writings. And Western medicine moved forward quickly with the writings of Hippocrates. Briefly, Hippocrates focused on a natural treatment approach to disease, as opposed to divine providence, which had, more often than not, been considered the cause of, and supported the basic treatment of, disease (Kleisiaris, Sfakianakis, and Papathanasiou, n.d.; see also Guthrie, Underwood, Richardson, Rhodes, and Thomson, 2019). Hippocrates, however, followed the school of Asclepieion medical practice, which had, as its "medical thinking model," a focus on maintaining the overall health and health status of the patient, as well as "natural" disease treatments from herbs and other plants. Furthermore, rather than blaming divine providence or spirits for diseases, Hippocrates and his disciples indicated that most illnesses had a specific and natural cause.

Hippocrates was also one of the first individuals who pointed out that food, nature, and climate could contribute to disease, while taking care of health could help combat it. It could be said that Hippocrates gave birth to the concept of preventative medicine, pointing out that physical activity was one way to strengthen the body, which, in turn, could ward off disease. Hippocrates also believed that mental illnesses could be treated more effectively if handled in a manner similar to physical medical decisions, involving the role of music and theater in treatment. Hippocrates also focused on medical conduct, which is what will be discussed later in this book.

In terms of any kind of disclosure, on the one hand, many

modern medical ethicists considered the Greek physician-patient relationship as paternalistic, meaning telling a patient the truth about illnesss or treatment wasn't necessarily part of medical treatment (Miles, 2009). On the other hand, the actual Hippocratic canon from the Cos school (which functioned at around 400 BCE) indicated the importance of honesty within the physician-patient relationship.

While the Hippocratic Oath itself says little about requiring physician disclosure, Hippocrates himself (or themselves, as some scholars believe "Hippocrates" was a singular name for a group of individuals) apparently supported the idea of disclosure and honesty. However, as the practice of medicine became more sophisticated and technologically focused, the process of any kind of medical disclosure, from either adverse events or diagnoses, became less likely.

## ◆ The Growing Cult of Secrecy: The Inability to Disclose

Sokol (2006) reminds us that the doctor-patient relationship was vastly different at the dawn of the twentieth century versus that at the dawn of the twenty-first. When the calendar flipped to 1900, the typical patient tolerated, and even expected, a medical tyranny that wouldn't be accepted today (see also Shorter, 1985). For one thing, practitioners weren't in the business of communicating much of anything to their patients (or families), even though, from an ethical standpoint, they might have been required to do so.

In fact, physician-patient communication began eroding as early as the seventeenth and eighteenth centuries, especially in the United States. Sisk et al. (2016) said that, for example, "disclosing bad news to patients has challenged physicians since the early days of American medicine." One book, written by D. W. Cathell in the early part of the eighteenth century, categorically stated that physicians shouldn't provide patients with tools to diagnose or treat themselves (Sisk, Frankel, Kodish, and Isaacson, 2016).

Furthermore, in the early days of the American Medical Association (specifically, during the mid-1800s), the organization's Code of Ethics specifically indicated that

> A physician should not be forward to make gloomy prognostications, because they savor of empiricism ... But he should not fail, on proper occasions, to give to the friends of the patient timely notice of danger, when it really occurs; and even to the patient himself, if absolutely necessary ... For, the physician should be the minister of hope and comfort to the sick. (Sisk, Frankel, Kodish, and Isaacson, 2016)

(See also *Code of Ethics of the American Medical Association*, 1847.)

At that time, the AMA suggested that physicians weren't under any obligation to disclose an ailment or potential death, as it was thought that such disclosure might harm the patient and cause him or her mental anguish.

Nor was it only the AMA that suggested its doctors move away from honest disclosure. John Gregory and Thomas Percival, both nineteenth-century doctors, considered "deception to be morally justified when used in the patient's best interests" (Sokol, 2006). This refusal to disclose especially included disclosure of medical errors—if an adverse event took place, doctors kept silent, and patients (and their families) didn't realize that such an event had taken place. The patient, ignorant of the disease or procedure, was kept in the dark if a mistake took place.

One reason for the increasing culture of secrecy, versus that of disclosure, was because of the doctor-patient relationship itself. Doctors were fast becoming the all-knowing experts of all sorts of diseases and their treatments, often treating their patients with condescension and paternalism. The patients, in turn, still baffled by the mysteries of medicine (and still believing in faith and divine providence as a cause of disease and potential cure), rarely crossed their doctors or questioned their diagnoses. Rather, they accepted them and didn't think to question the situation if something went wrong. As such, the doctor-patient relationship ended up resembling that of a parent and child; the doctors believed that patients didn't need to know everything, as such knowledge would end up harming them. It was this philosphy, in fact, that made up, and enforced, the AMA's initial Code of Ethics.

While paternalism and benevolence were the reason for the AMA's stance of (mostly) silence when it came to disclosure (or not disclosing, as the case was), other darker reasons were also in place. It's important to remember that even as medicine began leaving the Dark Ages in the eighteenth and nineteenth centuries, the field itself continued to be poorly organized, had limited authority, and offered even less in the way of education (Sisk, Frankel, Kodish, and Isaacson, 2016). Certainly, the first medical school in the United States opened in the mid-eighteenth century. However, medical schools were more an adjunct to, rather than a replacement for, education. The medical schools of today weren't as prevalent at that time; physicians were trained as apprentices, with little to no oversight as to quality of training. Doctors who made mistakes, leading to adverse events, didn't realize the fault might have been theirs.

As an example, throughout the 1800s and early 1900s, mercury was considered to be a remedy for everything from depression to syphillis. These days, we of course know that mercury is a heavy metal, which causes all kinds of ailments and eventually leads to death. This information was, however, not known at the time during which mercury was used as a medication. The fact that this substance was leading to muscle weakness, headaches, insomnia, and physical tremors didn't really gain traction until the mid-twentieth century. As such, doctors used the drug, believing it to be beneficial and putting the side effects down to other causes.

Furthermore, we also need to remember that eighteenth- and nineteenth-century physicians were far from the only game in town when it came to treatment of ailments. They were in competition with eclectics and homeopaths, not to mention "snake oil" salesmen. In the early days of US health care, the medicines available to physicians weren't a whole lot better than those available to snake oil salesmen or quacks. Medicine, overall, wasn't the respected profession it would become. As such, a physician admitting wrongdoing would be thought to put the industry in a poor light, adding insult to the injury that was disrespect for the profession (Sisk, Frankel, Kodish, and Isaacson, 2016).

As more helplful medications became available in the twentieth century and the practice of medicine became more sophisticated, the character and role of doctors also changed. Yet interestingly enough, adverse event disclosure didn't increase, nor did physician-patient communication. The growing class divide, combined with the perceived dangers of bad news, meant that physicians continued withholding important information from patients, whether that information consisted of diagnoses or adverse medical errors (Sisk, Frankel, Kodish, and Isaacson, 2016).

Noted one article from the late nineteenth century,

> In regard to cancer, the consensus of opinion is that patients be kept in ignorance of the nature and probable outcome of the disease as long as possible, in this way obviating the severe mental depression which invariably accompanies such knowledge. (Mapes, 1898)

The medical establishment didn't withhold information to be contrary. Rather, the belief was that disclosure would be a mental obstacle to a cure or could lead to a fatal shock. Bad news would be bad for the patient's mental health, it was thought. The less the patient knew about a particular situation or potential adverse event, the more confidence or hope that indiviudal would have, leading to a more positive outcome of treatment (Osler, 1909). And patients and their families, believing that nothing was wrong, continued to be blissfully unaware of either diseases or mistakes that might have been made in the treatment of such diseases.

Yet, this viewpoint and culture of silence had its detractors, most notably, the Reverand Thomas Gisborne, who indicated that lying to patients didn't do much good to inspire hope (Jackson, 2001). His belief was that patients who were very ill already knew they were ill and could see straight through the well-meaning lies of doctors' falsehoods.

While it might be easy to put the lack of disclosure down to the character of the medical profession of the 1700s and 1800s, the culture of diagnostic secrecy in American medicine continued well into the mid-twentieth century. As recently as 1961, 90 percent of physicians surveyed said they preferred not to disclose cancer diagnoses to patients (Oken, 1961). In fact, many said they would actively change the diagnosis to avoid any mention of cancer. In other words, practitioners admitted to outright lying when it came to sharing a diagnosis with a patient.

By this time, so much competition from quacks and lack of pharmaceuticals prompted the continued secrecy. The reason for continued nondisclosure ranged from the fact that physicians didn't get to know their patients well enough to judge desire for disclosure to ensuring that patients wouldn't create a scene in front of others when they were told the truth about a particular diagnosis or whether medical error was the cause of an adverse event (Glaser, 1966). In short, practitioners tended to underestimate the patients' abilitites to accept bad news when it came to health or disease.

The 1960s, however, began marking a change in the area of health care and disclosure. President Lyndon B. Johnson's "Great Society" brought about the expansion of Social Security to include Medicare and Medicaid; this, and other expansions under state and federal guidelines, meant the government assumed additional responsibility for the safety of its citizens. That safety meant a requirement of more honesty and clarification when it came to medical treatment and disease.

Alongside of this, well-publicized medical-related controversies, such as the Tuskegee study of untreated syphilis in black males came to light in the early 1970s (Waxman, 2017). The Tuskegee study, conducted in 1932, delibately injected black men with syphilis for "research" and then lied to them about treating the disease. This despicable study, which was only to have lasted for six months, actually lasted for more than forty years. The Associated Press broke the story about the study in 1972; the result was a perhaps unsurprising outcry. The issue here involved informed consent (there was none when it came to the study's participants). This, in turn, led to development of an advisory panel that concluded the study was unethically justified. The truth behind such studies led to a growing adversarial relationship between health-care practitioners and the public (Sisk, Frankel, Kodish, and Isaacson, 2016). No longer did patients treat their physicians like God but rather tended to be a little more cautious when accepting platitudes or falsehoods about their care and treatment. The upshot of growing knowledge was that by 1973, the American Hospital Association created "A Patient's Bill of Rights," which allowed that patients had a right to obtain "relevant, current and understandable information concerning diagnosis, treatment and prognosis" (AHA Patient's Bill of Rights, 1992). Several organizations created their own "Patient's Bill of Rights," but the gist of the matter was that patients had a right to understand what was going on when it came to any kind of medical care.

And, interstingly enough, physicians themselves began calling for more transparency when it came to sharing diagnoses and honest treatment with patients. A physicians' progressive movement, which started in the late 1960s, provided momentum when it came to better disclosure of patients' illnesses. As younger practitioners graduated from medical school and began to practice medicine, transparency and honesty became more of a given, with communication between physicians and patients more the norm than the exception (Sisk, Frankel, Kodish, and Isaacson, 2016).

This doesn't mean, however, that open and honest communication between physicians and patients is a 100 percent given, even today. For instance, a fairly recent report from the Alzheimer's Association indicated that less than half of patients with the disease—or their family members—had knowledge of the diagnosis ("Alzheimer's Disease: Facts and Figures," 2015).

And while physician/patient communication is better than it was even fifty years ago, we've already seen that doctors haven't always owned up to any medical errors or adverse events that might have occurred. In fact, it wasn't until the late 1990s that it was realized just how prevalent medical errors were and that anything needed to be done about it.

### ◆ To Err Is Human: Opening the Pandora's Box of Adverse Events

The first major study focused on adverse medical events in the United States took place in California during the early 1970s (Waite, 2005; see also Mills, 1977). The study noted that adverse events took place in 4.6 percent of all hospital admissions. While interesting, this particular study didn't necessarily raise any alarms.

After all, less than 5 percent of a medical population wasn't exactly newsworthy.

The same lack of interest held true with a Harvard medical practice study, which analyzed more than thirty thousand randomly selected medical charts of patients discharged from New York State hospitals. That study noted a high incidence of adverse events, indicating that such events occurred in 3.7 percent of hospitalizations (Brennan, et al., 1991). Somewhat more alarming was that 58 percent of the events were preventable, as 29 percent of them were due to negligence.

A similar study detailing Colorado and Utah hospitals, which noted that adverse events took place in 3 percent of hospitalizations in each state, and 54 percent of those were preventable (Gawande, Thomas, Zinner, and Brennan, 1999).

Yet, as mentioned earlier, these studies didn't necessarily raise any eyebrows. Even before the studies, few were ignorant enough to believe that doctors never made mistakes. What people didn't realize, however, was the scope and extent to which medical errors took place. This fact was blown wide opened with the Institute of Medicine's (IOM) November 1999 report *To Err Is Human: Building a Safer Health System* (Institute of Medicine, 1999). The report outlined specific medical errors (ranging from wrong-site surgery, to falls, to mistaken patient identities), pointing out that "high error rates with serious consequences are most likely to occur in intensive care units, operating rooms and emergency departments" (1999).

The report was researched and put together by the IOM's Committee on Quality Health Care in America, which had, as its focus, addressing patient safety as a key quality component

(Donaldson, 2008). *To Err Is Human* was originally conceived of as a quality document; the IOM's goal wasn't to call out specific health-care providers but rather to find ways in which errors could be reduced and quality care of patients be improved.

Yet the research put together by the IOM caused a great stir. In its report, the organization estimated that between 44,000 and 98,000 people died each year from a result of preventable medical error (Institute of Medicine, 1999). Improving the quality of health-care delivery, the report said, could help reduce the number of adverse medical events.

The report also put a cost figure on the toll of medical errors, pointing out that, between lost income, household productivity, and disability, such errors cost the nation between $17 billion and $29 billion per year in hospitals nationwide. Finally, the report pointed out that errors were leading to a loss of trust in the health-care system by patients, as well as diminished satisfaction by providers and other professionals.

Other interesting aspects of the report focused on the causes of such adverse medical events, which included the following:

- The decentralized and fragmented nature of health-care delivery, also dubbed as the "nonsystem"—noted the report, "When patients see multiple providers in different settings, none of whom has access to complete information, it becomes easier for things to go wrong."
- Licensure and accreditation have only a limited focus on medical error prevention, "and even these minimal efforts have confronted resistance from some health-care organizations and providers," the report said.

- Providers perceive the medical liability system as a "serious impedement" to focusing on efforts that would lead to uncovering and learning from medical errors.
- Third-party purchasers of health care (such as insurance companies) were providing little to no financial incentive for health-care organizations and providers to improve safety and quality.

The main conclusion of the report was that the majority of medical errors aren't necessarily the result of individual recklessness or ignorant practitioners. Rather, errors were taking place because of "faulty systems, processes, and conditions that lead people to make mistakes, or fail to present them," the report said. In other words, from the IOM's point of view, pointing fingers at doctors and other health-care providers for adverse events was counterproductive, because it was the system itself, as well as its many components, that was the basis of most adverse medical events.

The report concluded by offering a variety of strategies for improvement, which included the following:

- establishing a national focus on leadership, tools, and protocols to improve the patient safety knowledge base
- identifying and learning from errors, through development of a public mandatory reporting system and by encouraging health-care organizations and providers to participate in such voluntary reporting systems
- improving performance and safety standards through the actions of oversight organizations, professional groups, and health-care purchasers

- implementation of safety systems in health-care organizations, to ensure safe practices at the delivery level

The sheer scope of the report, and its conclusions, did catch the attention of the public and media. The idea, especially, that up to 98,000 patients died because of medical errors was certainly newsworthy. One immediate response to the IOM report included the 2001 Joint Commission on the Accreditation of Hospital Organizations requirement that all unanticipated outcomes be communicated to patients or their families (Taft, 2005; see also LeGros and Pinkall, 2002).

Nor was it just health-care systems that were singled out in *To Err Is Human*. The legal system and its impact on medicine was also highlighted, with the IOM pointing out that lawsuits and malpractice filings weren't effective when it comes to recompensation for injured patients (Institute of Medicine, 1999; see also Liebman and Hyman, 2004).

Another response was that of potential legislation. In late 2005, Senators Hillary Clinton (D-NY) and Barack Obama (D-IL) introduced the National Medical Error Disclosure and Compensation Act (MEDiC), which encouraged the medical community to adopt a policy of full medical error disclosure (Kaiser, 2006). The act was to have created an Office of Patient Safety and Health Care Quality, which has established a national patient safety database. While the bill didn't make it out of the Senate committee, the document's key provisions ended up being published in the *New England Journal of Medicine* (Tan, 2015). Furthermore, the bill was also in line with many of the "apology laws" passed by several state legislatures.

Since *To Err Is Human* was released in 1999, there has been more transparency when it comes to admitting medical error. There are many, however, who believe we are still a long way from acknowledging adverse events—and learning from them. In a guest editorial in *Nursing Critical Care*, Anne Marie Palatnik (2016) pointed out that "unfortuantely, we have not come close to achieving the IOM's goal," in other words, that of ensuring patient safety through health-care systems improvement or even disclosure. She pointed out that in 2013, approximately 400,000 people died from preventable medical errors. "To have a culture of safety," she added, "there must be transparency, mutual trust and an environment that promotes learning from errors."

One factor getting in the way of transparency, trust, and learning is the current reaction to many adverse medical events, which is the malpractice lawsuit. As such, to understand the deny-and-defend culture of medicine and disclosure of adverse medical events, it's important to understand the impact of the law on the practice of medicine.

### ◆ Legal Briefs: The Link between Medicine and the Law

The connection between medicine and the law is a long one, going back thousands of years (Anderson, 2017). The earliest mention of repercussions for medical error is, once again, in Hammurabi's Code. As mentioned earlier, the code indicated that a doctor could be severely punished if harm was done to a patient. Such punishment could be as severe as cutting off the doctor's hands, if the doctor killed the patient (Guthrie, Underwood, Richardson, Rhodes, and Thomson, 2019). This probably explained why doctors in Hammurabi's time weren't too anxious to disclose wrongdoing.

Roman law also recognized medical malpractice as a legal wrong (Kass and Rose, 2016). While harming physicians for wrongdoing wasn't as prevelant, Roman law still was punitive if medical treatment went awry.

The idea of legal remedies for medical malpractice found its way to Europe during the thirteenth century CE. Malpractice was also widely accepted, as theory, in the English legal system (Wallace, 2017). In 1768, Sir William Blackstone tied the concept of liability to physicians, pointing out that injuries due to neglect or unskillful management of a patient were grounds for suit.

Malpractice ultimately came to the United States from England. The first malpractice case mentioned in America took place in 1794, in which a plaintiff claimed that a doctor had promised to conduct a skillful operation but instead did the opposite, with the plaintiff's wife dying as a result (Anderson, 2017). The plaintiff won the case, perhaps setting the stage for a way in which patients could obtain some recompense for errors. Throughout the 1800s, the United States experienced an increase in medical malpractice cases.

As medical technology grew in the pratice of medicine throughout the nineteenth century, complications from treatments became more frequent. Once such technology—that of anesthesia use for surgeries and other procedures—became the leading cause of medical malpractice litigation throughout the 1800s (Wallace, 2017). This is because early anesthesiologists were guessing when it came to the actual amount of the drug to be administered to render a patient unconscious, which often led to death or impairment.

Interestingly enough, as lawsuits increased, a few leading American physicians in the first part of the nineteenth century actually encouraged such legal action, pointing out that "in an era of often very questionable medical practitioners ... patient safety would be enhanced by ... lawsuits."

It probably should come as little surprise that physician support of legal redress for medical errors diminished in the twentieth century, as numerous reforms were passed, with courts publishing standards of medical malpractice awards. This ended up boosting the amount of awards, many times, into the millions of dollars, though state and federal laws were passed to cap certain amounts of certain types of damages.

Even in this day and age of our litigious society, it shouldn't be assumed that patients have an easy road when it comes to suing a practitioner for a treatment gone awry. From a legal standpoint, if an injured party wants to prevail in a medical malpractice suit against a health-care provider, the plaintiff needs to indicate that the following four elements are present (Kass and Rose, 2016):

- The physician had a duty to the patient.
- The physician was negligent in his or her execution of the duty.
- The physician's negligence was the proximate cause of the patient's injury.
- The patient's injury resulted in damages.

According to *To Err Is Human*, the court is really no place for admission of medical error. Liability is very costly and can take years to resolve; many times, such suits don't make it as far as a trial by jury. Yet in many ways (and as Beth Daley Ullem learned), a lawsuit can be the only way to break the culture of secrecy that can hide disclosure of medical error. It's safe to say that because of the high cost of litigation, doctors are in fear that if they admit any kind of wrongdoing, a patient—or the patient's family—might respond with a slew of lawyers. Later on in this book, I'll discuss why disclosure doesn't necessarily lead to legal action. I'll also explain how malpractice litigation is exactly the wrong way to encourage disclosure.

But first, it's important to understand the ethical duty that a physician has when it comes to disclosing information to a patient.

# THE ETHICS OF PHYSICIAN DISCLOSURE

THE ETHICAL ARGUMENT IS STRAIGHTFORWARD WHEN it comes to disclosing information to patients. Namely, patients have the right to know everything about their care, and hospitals don't have a legal or moral right to withhold the information (Leape, 2012). Despite this, however, disclosure isn't always forthcoming, even in this day and age, when the relationship between doctors and patients has moved from, as Sokol put it, "unquestioning acquiescence" to a partnership where patients have an authorative voice in decision-making, leading to more truthful disclosures (Sokol, 2006).

But how much should a physician actually disclose to a patient? Certainly, "first do no harm" has been a foundation of medicine for millennia (Waite, 2005). Harm committed with the intent of healing is prohibited by the principle of nonmaleficence as much as malicious harm might be. This could also focus on harm done to a patient by keeping silent.

Overall, the personal duties of the physician must focus on the following:

- practicing with veracity
- honoring patient autonomy when managing medical situations
- ensuring informed consent for procedures
- enhancing human flourishing
- promoting the common good and social justice
- maintaining beneficence and nonmaleficence
- curbing paternalism
- ensuring respect for people/patients/families
- maintaining a patient's right to privacy

While some of these could be found in Hippocrates's time, they mainly evolved over time. Honesty and virtue, however, could be found in the philosophies of many ancient ethicists.

## ◆ Obligation to Disclose: The Philosophers of Ancient Greece

What's interesting is that googling "medical error disclosure" or "disclosure of adverse medical events" and "Greek philosophers" doesn't bring up specific articles or statements. Other than Hippocrates, who certainly focused on the rights and wrongs of health care, there is not too much available that specifically ties disclosure to the practice of medicine. However, there is plenty of information out there linking ancient and historical philosophers with medical ethics, in general. To that end, this section will focus on what some of these more famous philosophers had to say about medical ethics and doctor-patient relationships and then extrapolate those issues to the disclosure of adverse events.

The ancient Greek philosphers worked hard to tie together virtue and happiness (*Stanford Encyclopedia of Philosophy*, 2014). In other words, the more "virtuous" an individual proved to be, the happier he or she would likely be.

Starting out with Socrates, his writings in the "Apology" point out that "a man worth anything at all does not reckon whether his course of action endangers his life or threatens death." He was a philosopher who placed moral considerations above all others, with justice being considered as a way in which others are treated. His collection of unjust actions included robbing temples, betraying friends, stealing, breaking oaths, committing adultry, and mistreating parents. He also points out that virtue (which guarantees "good" action) is knowledgeable, as well as being sufficient for happiness. The Socratic philosophy doesn't directly discuss any kind of medical ethics or the need to disclose medical mistakes, but it does introduce the concept of justice, which his student, Plato, carried on. Socrates's philosophy was that honesty was good and betrayal was bad. As such, we could probably note that withholding a diagnosis or medical error could be a sign of "dishonesty," or at the very least was not ethical.

Meanwhile, Socrates's student Plato used on dialogues, based on his teacher's philosophies. These too focused on the notion of morality (*Stanford Encyclopedia of Philosophy*, 2014). Specificially (and "speaking through" Socrates), Plato explains that moral psychology is an account of the soul that, in turn, is a basis for supporting and explaining virtue (*Stanford Encyclopedia of Philosophy*, 2014). He also introduces the concept of reason, which is basically considered as "what is good both for oneself and in the treatment of others" (*Stanford Encyclopedia of Philosophy*, 2014).

When it comes to Plato (and his Socratic writings), Lidz (1995) explains that the philosopher's writings frequently rely on medical metaphor. For instance, a character's condition and ethical behavior require development and care, as does a healthy body. Plato's focus emphasizes prevention rather than cure and focuses on intellectual regimes for optimal health (Lidz, 1995). The other implication is that moral condition is inward, as is health—the focus here is on character and ensuring that observation of one's present actions are conducive to health (Lidz, 1995). Furthermore, according to Plato, as doctors can vary in levels of competence, so do people; people who might have a greater moral ability will likely demand more of themselves than someone of lesser moral ability (Lidz, 1995). In other words, what is right or appropriate for one person might not be right or appropriate for another (Lidz, 1995). Translating this to disclosure of errors, Plato seems to be taking an "it depends" stance. In other words, disclosing medical errors might not be the right choice to make in all situations, even as not all individuals will operate at the same level of moral functioning.

Overall, when it came to caring for a patient, it seems as though Plato did accept withholding of information, because such disclosure wasn't always right or correct for specific patients (Sokol, 2006).

Then, there was Artistotle and his focus on justice. Aristotle indicated that justice is responsible for promoting the common interest (Cohen-Almagor, 2017). The concept of Aristotle's justice when it comes to health care discussed mostly allocation of resources; in other words, how those resources were allocated depended on patients' states of health and how likely they were to survive. However, Aristotle's belief also points out that moral responsibility is a part of virtue ethics. Basically, from Aristotle's point of view, "a moral individual is one who strives for excellence and virtuous living ... an individual can be considered a person of integrity if her character, decisions and actions are congruent with virtuous behavior."

The question here is whether disclosing a medical error is virtuous behavior, at least, from Aristotle's point of view. The answer would be, it depends on that doctor's responsibility to that patient. Aristotle defines responsible physicians as those who can understand the consequences of their choice, or action—they "are able to appreciate likely consequences of a given conduct." In other words, it could be said, from the Aristolean point of view, that disclosing an adverse medical event would be the moral and right thing to do, as long as the doctor understands the consequences of the behavior, both good and bad. If that action is likely to harm the patient, then disclosure would not take place.

Examining the ancient philosophers' viewpoints toward disclosure, in general, is a mixed bag. Certainly, there is the morality and justice inherent with disclosure. However, there is also the question as to whether disclosure of all events is a necessity.

Narrowing this down to the disclosure of adverse medical events to a patient, applying ancient Greek teachings to this question doesn't yield a clear yes or no answer. Rather, such honesty and disclosure likely depend on the situation. While honesty is moral and just, disclosure might not be the best possible scenario for a patient, at least, according to the ancient Greeks.

## ◆ Hippocrates: Foggy Approach to Error Disclosure

While we can only extrapolate how the ancient Greek philosophers might view medical ethics or the ethics behind medical disclosure, we have much more information when it comes to Hippocrates and his view toward ethics and medicine. What's interesting is that the main thrust of the Hippocratic Oath—"First, do no harm"—doesn't specifically appear in the oath itself (Berdine, 2015). Rather, that phrase was attributed to Thomas Sudenham, a British phyisician in the seventeenth century.

The original Hippocratic Oath in fact focused extensively on four parts: a pledge to pagan dieties, a list of positive obligations, a list of negative obligations, and a statement of piety. I'm examining these four parts in depth, as it provides a good basis on which the original Hippocratic Oath (and the doctors who took it) operated.

### *Pledge to Pagan Dieties*

It needs to be remembered that ancient Greece was a polythestic society (in other words encompassing many gods as part of the daily religious rituals), and this particular part of the oath focused on pledges to Apollo, among others. This is because divine-command theory was the basis of ancient ethical systems, with the differences between right and wrong determined through deity commands. Basically, "a pledge to a deity is equivalent to a pledge to act morally right."

## List of Positive Obligations

These requirements included honoring teachers; professional courtesy (in that no physician typically charges another physician for services); working to aid patients, according to the physician's ability and judgment (with the first duty to the patient); and nonmaleficence (Berdine, 2015). This latter focuses on keeping patients from harm and injustice and was the basis of the "do no harm" clause with which today's patients and physicians are familiar.

Berdine indicated that more modern ethics under this particular category could be based on utilitarianism, in other words, the greatest good should be generated for the greatest number of people. Such a system requires a great deal of thought, comparing advantages and disadvantages of each particular action and then determining the decision that will offer the best possible outcome to the most people. Berdine uses the concept of vaccines as an example. Vaccines do offer the benefit of herd immunity but can also carry unwanted side effects. The physician must determine if the greater good of herd immunity outweighs those side effects.

If we focus on this concept of medical error disclosure, we have the same issue. While disclosure of adverse events might provide the greater good for many people, it could also provide harm to both the patient (who might not want to know), the patient's family, and the physician, who might end up with angry patients, at best, or a lawsuit, at worst. This fear, by the way, continues with the culture of secrecy focus I'll be detailing later on in this book.

### List of Negative Obligations

The negative obligations in Hippocrates's original oath included prohibitions against euthanasia, abortion, sexual relations with patients, protecting guild turf (for example, physicians won't act as surgeons), and adherence to confidentiality.

### Concluding Piety

This statement was a pledge amounting to the idea that if the physician violated any of the preceding sections of the oath, his or her life could be hellish. Berdine pointed out that this final section is "a common literary device for a pledge" and is seen in a lot of oaths.

What is interesting to note is that the Hippocratic Oath, then and these days, while focused on doing no harm, doesn't necessarily focus on telling the truth to patients (or keeping the truth from them). Other things the Hippocratic Oath doesn't support include honoring patient preferences, sharing medical information with patients, protecting patients who enroll in research studies, avoiding the practice of medicine while impaired, and avoiding conflicts of interest (Shmerling, 2015).

And while the Hippocratic Oath is considered the foundation and basis of modern medicine, the oath, in and of itself, isn't necessarily used any more when it comes to modern physicians. One study pointed out that barely half of US medical schools administered the oath upon graduation, while only 2 percent of the institutions used the oath in its original form. Another survey among practicing physicians indicated that while 80 percent of those questioned reported participating in an oath ceremony, only a quarter felt that the oath affected how they practiced.

Getting back to ancient Greece, Hippocratic writings encouraged doctors to be sparing with the truth and not reveal anything about the patient's future or present condition and whether the patient was in any shape to receive information about their medical conditions (Sokol, 2006).

It seems as though Greek physicians took this advice to heart. On the one hand, in Hippocrates's day, physicians seemed to be in favor of sharing information about adverse events from medical treatment with other physicians, namely because such sharing helped improve the practice of medicine (Miles, 2004). However, when it came to sharing that information with a patient or relative, the situation was markedly different. According to Miles, "none of the dozens of accounts of errors in the ancient Green texts advocates or illustrates telling a patient or relative about an error." The reason for this was because Greek physicians were afraid of being unfairly accused of the error and were sensitive when it came to being accused of error. That fear of reaction to disclosure of an adverse medical event seems to be driving the reason behind withholding such information, even to this day.

To conclude this section about the ancient Greeks' attitudes toward medical ethics, we focus on the theory of ethics and the reality about what actually (likely) took place. In theory, the Greek philosophers supported justice, fairness, and truth. But Hippocrates, the "father of medicine," supported this only to an extent.

The question brought up by the ancient Greek philosophers was the concept of moral rightness. In most cases, such "rightness" depended on an individual's point of view. As such, when it came to the disclosure of medical errors, ancient Greek physicians not only had to determine what they believed, in their hearts, was morally right but also what would be right for the physician. Hippocrates tended to support the point of view of silence in the face of adverse events, at least silence when it came to sharing negative information with the patient. Given the fear of being blamed for any kind of adverse medical event, Greek physicians often felt patient silence was the right way to go, though confessing errors to other physicians was certainly allowed and encouraged, in an effort to help provide an overall benefit to the practice of medicine. There was no patient's bill of rights during the time of Hippocrates and, likely as not, no need or desire to disclose information to the patient.

### ◆ Ethical Models Today

Fast-forwarding to today, however, physicians and ethicists seem to agree, in theory, that disclosure to a patient is necessary in most cases. We know that the patient's bill of rights requires full disclosure of an error and diagnosis to patients (Ghazai, Saleem, and Amlani, 2014). Delving into this further, we see that the patient's bill of rights can take many forms. The following is an example of some clauses in a bill of rights, as outlined by the National Institutes of Health Clinical Center (2019). It includes mandates such as

- The patient is to receive safe, considerate, and respectful care, provided in a manner that is consistent with the patient's beliefs.

- Records and communication pertaining to treatment will be treated as confidential.
- The patient is to receive complete information about diagnosis, treatment, and prognosis from the practitioner, in terms that are easily understood.
- The patient is to receive information necessary for the patient to give informed consent, prior to any procedure or treatment.

And when it comes to ethics, health-care practitioners are bound by the principles of beneficence and nonmaleficence. Beneficence in medical practice refers to avoiding and preventing error by doing well, while nonmaleficence focuses on avoiding harm to oneself and others, whenever possible. Under these auspices, it could be considered that holding back on an error can cause grave harm to the patient, as failure to disclose an adverse medical event can end up making a bad situation worse (Edwin, 2009). I mentioned earlier that many patients understand that they might be seriously ill, even if a doctor indicates otherwise. As such, beneficence mandates honesty and truth-telling, because the patient might be in a position in which he or she is worrying needlessly about a worsening condition, thinking it might be part of an underlying disease, rather than the result of medical error in the course of treatment. An understanding that what is going on could be the result of a medical error could prevent psychological distress from negatively affecting a patient's condition. This flies in the face of the idea that withholding information from the patient is a good thing, as knowing bad news could adversely harm the individual.

Beneficence, furthermore, means physicians are required to remove any condition that will harm others (as well as prevent harm from occuring to others). Returning to the task of medical disclosure, beneficence conveys a moral obligation on the physician to act for the benefit of others. In this situation, the act of beneficence focuses on prevention and removal of harms. Within this parameter, "disclosure of error to the patient will enhance the trust in the physician ... (while) disclosure to the hospital management will help to improve processes and reduce errors for the future." Doing the opposite, in other words, failing to disclose a medical error that has taken place—and letting the patient assume that what he or she is going through is the result of the disease or condition—is unkind, harmful, and violates the principle of beneficence.

Furthermore, errors of omission (in other words, not disclosing an error if a patient doesn't ask about it) are also considered highly unethical and deceptive. This falls under the principle of autonomy, a scenario that encourages the patient's right to have full information about treatments and any mistakes that might have occurred. Under the concept of autonomy, the patient requires full information about a specific situation in order to make the best decision possible when it comes to moving forward.

Additionally, if a physician doesn't disclose an error to a patient, he or she places his or her own interest above that of the patient, "thereby violating a patient-centered ethic." The practitioner is thinking about him- or herself and what the consequences of disclosure might be to his or her own standing, rather than what's actually in the patient's best interests.

Finally, there is the ethical consideration of justice, which, in this case, can be defined as "fair, equitable and appropriate treatment in light of what is due, or owed, to persons." As I pointed out earlier, the ancient Greek philsophers set a great deal of store in justice. Furthermore, by its very nature, the principle of justice dictates error disclosure, in an effort to provide appropriate compensation to patients. The result of a medical error could be increased health costs and lost wages, meaning compensation would be necessary to help defray some of these costs. Knowing about a medical error can enable patients to obtain necessary compensation, which can range from receiving monies for lost income or obtaining a discount on the medical bill.

To conclude, while ancient philosophers might have been somewhat wishy-washy when it comes to physician disclosure to patients, the more modern-day ethicists are fairly adamant that honesty is the best policy. Specifically, physicians have the duty to disclose anything, and everything that might result in an adverse scenario when it comes to patient treatment.

# MEDICINE, APOLOGIES, AND LITIGATION: THE PRESENT

IN THEORY, PHILOSOPHERS AND ETHICISTS BELIEVE THAT physician disclosure is a positive thing and should be a requirement when it comes to patients. In the preceding section, I noted that the practice of medicine, in and of itself, requires respect for patient autonomy, as well as removing harm and doing no harm. As such, disclosure can be considered an important part of medical care.

Certainly, modern-day ethicists endorse full medical error disclosure to patients. And, far from wanting to avoid a worst-case scenario, patients want to be told when a medical error has occurred and want to be provided with detailed information regarding the nature of the error, why it happened, and what will be done to prevent future incidences from happening (Waite, 2005; see also Gallagher et al., 2003).

However, and perhaps, unfortunately, the response when it comes to adverse medical events and their disclosure tends to be buried in the concept of deny-and-defend.

### ◆ Deny-and-Defend: A Culture of Secrecy

Deny-and-defend occurs when an adverse event takes place and the patient or patient's family is not made aware of that event. The concept behind this procedure represents the medical establishment's attempt to repudiate culpability for wrongdoing (whether intentional or unwitting) and to defend procedures and the reasons the actions have taken place (Smith, 2019).

During the time of Hammurabi, there was a reason for a physician's denial; admitting to wrongdoing could likely lead to unpleasant consequences for the practitioner. And the practice of medicine during the eighteenth and nineteenth centuries also embraced disclosure, more because the practice of medicine wasn't accepted by all the population as a good thing. It's curious, however, that in this day and age, deny-and-defend continues to be the practice of the day.

While not all adverse events necessarily require full disclosure (which would be very difficult, if not impossible), deny-and-defend has, for the most part, been the standard approach to poor outcomes and adverse medical events (Welch, 2011). Deny-and-defend, basically, has been a way of protecting medical establishments from error and unanticipated outcomes, while throwing up an opaque wall against patients and their families who simply want to know the truth about why a particular medical procedure or course of treatment went wrong. The theory also goes that deny-and-defend is ideal in protecting doctors from costly lawsuits while absolving them of wrongdoing.

While health-care institutions, hospitals, risk managers, and attorneys believe that deny-and-defend is ideal when it comes to protecting the medical establishment from finger-pointing and potential wrongdoing, in truth, the concept creates a vicious cycle that not only keeps patients in the dark but also blocks information from coming out to prevent similar errors from taking place.

Specifically, here are the downfalls from the deny-and-defend model:

1) A lack of transparency in the face of an adverse medical event doesn't give the patient—or his or her family—necessary information when it comes to how that mistake occurred (Boothman, Blackwell, Campbell Jr., Commiskey, and Anderson, 2009; see also Sage, 2004). A lack of such information can lead to frustration, especially as the patient and his or her family only want to know the truth of a situation.
2) The continued lack of information and continued stonewalling by the health-care institution can, more often than not, lead to litigation, as the patient attempts to determine what went wrong and why. The problem, however, is that, with liability insurers who represent individual physicians either defending or settling most claims, it's likely that the patient or his or her family likely won't ever know what went wrong and why the adverse event took place (Sage, 2004).
3) During the process of a long, drawn-out lawsuit, physicans and providers continue to be cautioned to silence by insurance companies and hospital/physical counsel. They are also told to continually deflect responsibility, while making the legal process as slow, expensive, and drawn-out as possible for

plaintiffs to continue their fight and focus. As such, claims that involve serious injury can drag on for years—and, as information about the cause of injuries is denied to patients and their families for long periods of time, compensation isn't available when needed and qualilty feedback to providers is, more often than not, nonexistent. This raises frustration on the side of the patients and their families, who continue to lack information.

4) Such delay also means that malpractice insurance becomes more expensive. This is because the assumption is that a drawn-out case will be more expensive, meaning premiums will automatically be increased. This can create a hardship for the health-care provider, which, in turn, can also escalate care and overall health-care insurance costs and premiums.

5) If a malpractice suit actually gets as far as a trial, a decision either for the plaintiff (patient/family) or defendant (the physician) can be devastating. If the decision rules in favor of the plaintiff, it means the physician was in the wrong, which can be problematic for that individual's reputation and emotional well-being. Furthermore, it ensures that the reasons behind the error, in the first place, are not addressed, which means similar errors can take place in the future, with another potential costly and futile litigation process.

And if a decision is ruled in favor of the physician, the plaintiff is out of several thousand of dollars in legal fees and health-care expenses. To top it off, the plaintiff hasn't received any satisfaction or reasons why the error took place in the first place, thus adding to emotional anguish, frustration, and anger.

Deny-and-defend is in place at the expense of creating a climate in which patient safety is a priority (Boothman, Imhoff, and Campbell Jr., 2012). There is a reason, therefore, that Bootman, et al. dub deny-and-defend "a self-perpetuating spiral, that suppresses consideration of alternative approaches." Boothman and his colleagues went so far as to develop the following chart as an example of the negative outcomes of a deny-and-defend culture and system.

| Deny-and-Defend Elements | Outcomes |
|---|---|
| No apologies/information for an adverse event | Insurance companies pay more for mistakes and additional medical care required |
| Little or no explanation from physicians | Malpractice premiums rise |
| Keeping patients in the dark | Patients receive less compensation |
| Adversarial relationship | Attorneys earn the money |
| Increasing legal costs | Nothing is learned |
| Stressed physicians, burnout | More errors, errors are repeated |
| Frustrated patients and families | More patients are harmed |

Though risk managers and lawyers might believe the opposite, patients who experience adverse health-care events don't want to hire attorneys or go through the hassle of a lawsuit. They don't want to go through the expense of litigation or the possibility of needing to bring a trial to court. Doing so is expensive, time-consuming, and exhausting, and, unless there is a sure outcome in favor of the plaintiff, can end up burying the patient in legal fees without any kind of recompense or satisfaction for the investment of time and money.

So why do patients go through the time and trouble of litigation? In truth, patients, or their families, hire lawyers because they have little, if any, knowledge about the adverse event that caused either the death or disability of themselves or a loved one. Deny-and-defend ensures that information is secure and that patients are stonewalled by the institutions that are supposed to be overseeing their medical care (or the care of their loved ones). As such, those who experience medical errors and their outcomes often don't have all the facts as to what led to the adverse event in the first place. Additionally, those patients and families don't have the medical knowledge to make sense of what happened. Added to this is that caregivers and hospitals rarely, if ever, act to correct patients' or families' misconceptions about what went wrong or to correct their misunderstanding. This leads to more confusion and more frustration—such emotional scenarios don't benefit the patient in any way, shape, or form. In fact, it's the opposite; it could create harm, which is against the overall medical credo.

So, to conclude, deny-and-defend, which is in place in most medical institutions, even in this day in which patients and physicians are supposed to be partners, ensures that no one—not the patients or their attorneys—have access to the correct information in the face of an adverse medical event (Boothman, et al.). Furthermore, deny-and-defend has proven to be expensive and time-consuming, while doing little to nothing to correct the health-care system or to assuage a patient's fear or anger. Rather, this concept has developed, despite patient expectations and the physician's sense of his or her ethical duties, and is more the exception, than the norm, when it comes to dealing with adverse medical events (Boothman, Blackwell, Campbell Jr., Commiskey, and Anderson, 2009).

If deny-and-defend is so injurious to the health-care situation as well as patients (when simply disclosing the error could ensure this could be avoided), why is it in place?

Multiple factors can be blamed for the deny-and-defend mindset (Boothman, Imhoff, and Campbell Jr., 2012; see also Boothman, Blackwell, Campbell Jr., Commiskey, and Anderson, 2009). Some of the reasons are listed in the following.

### 1) *A fingerpointing health-care culture*

When a patient is injured in the course of a medical error or adverse event, medical institutions can take the stance of fight-or-blame. Typically, "morbidity and mortality" panels do take place in the face of a medical mistake resulting in injury or death to a patient, but such panels are focused more toward what happened and, in many cases, can focus on blame to the physician, nurses, or other providers, rather than correcting the error so it doesn't happen again. In such cases, hospitals and health-care systems can spend more time avoiding culpability and throwing practitioners under the bus for mistakes made than taking a clear-eyed look at the causes of the error and taking steps to address the error so it won't take place again.

### 2) *System failure*

At one time, medical error could be placed at the feet of a single physician or a group of physicians. However, in this day and age, health care can be delivered by many different providers (Gallagher, et al., 2013). As mentioned earlier, a system breakdown can cause adverse events—and while existing guidelines do provide focus on error disclosure, what is lacking is guidance on disclosing others' mistakes. Putting this in more simple terminology, doctors don't want to rat on their colleagues, if such a thing can be avoided. In such a scenario, health-care colleagues can close ranks, out of fear that telling the truth about an adverse medical event perpetrated by one physician or nurse could spell trouble for them, as well, in the future.

### 3) *Flight-or-fight reflexes*

The health-care community is, as Boothman et al. (2012) puts it, "hardwired, as all humans with a fight-or-flight reflex" when it comes to perceived danger or threats. This the case not just with the medical community. If someone makes a mistake, the first response is to sweep the error under the rug and not tell anyone about it. Make no mistake; when a physician makes a mistake that can cause injury, disability, or death, that flight-or-fight reflex can kick in. The difference between an average human being who errs and a physician who makes a mistake is that the latter is more often than not part of an organization with a vested interest in covering that mistake up. The reason for this is the fear of potential of lawsuits or litigation. Cover-ups (or "flight") can be regarded as the best and most prudent way for an institution to respond to a patient's complaints or to a patient's request for disclosure following an adverse medical event. The end result is similar to the one with which I introduced in this book; a patient's family member is left grieving because of a loss, and the health-care institution doesn't do anything to alleviate that grief with specific answers but rather is in a position to go ahead and continue making the same mistakes with the same results.

In addition, the medical community, more often than not, views a complaint or even an adverse medical event as a threat to its very foundation, rather than an opportunity to reach an understanding, based on communication, honesty, and openness. Deny-and-defend denies communication and the facts, preferring, instead, to remain behind secrecy, even when honesty might result in a decrease in litigation.

This leads us to the following point:

### 4) *The malpractice industry/advice of legal counsel*

Deny-and-defend has been spurred, to a great extent, by the malpractice insurance industry. Rather than urging disclosure in the aftermath of an adverse medical event, attorneys warn physicians that patients and families could view an apology or acknowledgment of an error as an admission of guilt, even when a physician is attempting to show compassion and remorse (Welch, 2011). Once a lawsuit is filed, trial lawyers, many times, don't help in this regard either. These attorneys also warn their physician clients that any admission of error during the litigation process could find its way into evidence, resulting in an adverse verdict. As a result, physicians and their health-care establishments are drawn, more and more, toward the trial lawyers' instinct to defend assigned claims by keeping silent and not saying anything that could compromise litigation, even if doing so might help defuse the situation at hand (Boothman, et al.). Basically, physicians, health-care providers, and health-care executives are advised not to talk about adverse events with patients or families, taken in by the idea (from risk managers and in-house counsel) that to do so would create problems, at best, and lead to costly ligitation, the ruining of their reputation, and career destruction, at worst. As we'll see later on in the book, the opposite is actually true. However, the fear of litigation continues to drive secrecy when it comes to medical institutions.

With such ligitation managed by a health-care system's risk managers or internal corporate lawyers, the trial lawyers' perspectives and advice (sue, sue, sue) go unchallenged and unregarded. Basically, in-house counsel and risk managers are all too ready to believe and take the advice of the trial lawyers, who might not have the best interests of the institution at heart.

### 5) *Disclosure discomfort*

When we make a mistake, we feel terrible about the action and its consequences. There is a reason why none of us want to acknowledge wrongdoing; otherwise, we would be doing so more often. Having to own up to our error is not a comfortable process. From our point of view, making that mistake makes us less than good people, and we like to convince ourselves that we are, indeed, good people. This type of emotional response to making a mistake is bad enough for people who don't carry the power of life and death in their hands—in other words, who aren't physicians. It goes without saying that physicians are responsible for the successful care and treatment of others. When that treatment goes awry and damages occur, the guilt of being the cause of that situation can be enormous.

Having to confess that guilt and wrongdoing to others can lead to disclosure discomfort—in other words, disclosing a mistake can lead to even more discomfort than created by the original error. For some who suffer from extreme disclosure discomfort, not having to talk to patients or their families about mistakes (because deny-and-defend prevents any kind of honest disclosure) can be almost a relief to the health-care provider, who simply wants it all to go away.

The problem with disclosure discomfort and the silence that it generates, however, is that it can be taken as dishonesty. No one likes the silent treatment when trying to find the facts of a situation. The fact that an organization is complicit in silence only creates additional distrust among patients and their families who have been wronged.

### 6) *Patient distress*

While medical ethical models support the idea of disclosure of an adverse event, doctors can refrain from disclosing such an event because doing so could cause the patient more emotional distress (Edwin, 2009). This is something we saw when it came to the ethics put forward by the ancient Greek philosophers, as well as the practice of early medical doctors. In this particular scenario, the physician might believe that not holding back information from disclosure would actually undermine a patient's automony, such as incapacitating an already severely depressed patient or sharing information with a patient who simply doesn't want to know what is going on. The argument here is that, if a medical error is disclosed, patients are likely to become more distressed about the error in question than they would be had they simply remained ignorant with the end result possibly being severely compromised care. If a doctor tells him- or herself that keeping something from a patient can be more beneficial, so the patient doesn't become emotional upon disclosure, that said physician is, in his or her own mind, upholding the principles of nonmaleficence and beneficence.

The truth, however, is that even if patients are distressed upon learning of a medical error, this is not a reason to keep it from them. Certainly, a patient might become angry when it comes to learning about the error, but it doesn't mean that the ability of that individual to make rational decisions would be at risk. Furthermore, while patients have described emotional responses following disclosure of medical errors (such as sadness, anxiety, and depression), many believe that their responses were less about the error itself and more about the manner in which it was disclosed. In other words, patients indicated that they would have been less upset if an error was disclosed honestly and compassionately; however, their frustration and distress tended to increase when error explanations were evasive or incomplete. As such, "patient distress" isn't a reason for nondisclosure, especially as such distress in the wake of disclosure tends to be more about the method of delivery as opposed to acknowledgment of the specific error.

To summarize, the culture of medical practice itself tends to lead to a focus on deny-and-defend when it comes to adverse medical events. Noted Lehman (2008), "the institution of medicine has created an entirely separate and mostly unspoken culture built around secrecy and non-disclosure."

Deny-and-defend aside, it can be hugely difficult for a practitioner to acknowledge wrongdoing. I mentioned disclosure discomfort earlier. But physicians are driven by more than simply being uncomfortable when admitting mistakes, which doesn't help when it comes to redressing the problem of acknowledging medical error.

### ◆ Sorry, Not Sorry: Practitioners and Difficult Apologies

As I mentioned in the opening of this book, mistakes are a fact of life in most industries; if a mistake is made, then the person responsible for the error apologizes, explains why the error took place, promises that steps will be taken so it doesn't happen again, and then offers the wronged person some sort of compensation. Most of us understand that saying, "I'm sorry," can go a long way toward righting a wrong. But when it comes to health care, as we've seen so far, the institution itself, from ancient times, tends to operate within secrecy and denial of culpability, rather than with openness and honesty.

When defense attorney Rick Boothman, described as the "father of the communication and resolution program," first introduced the University of Michigan model of medical error and disclosure (which I will discuss in more detail later on in this book) at a "Leading Medical Reform" conference in 2004, the result wasn't too good (Smith, 2019). At one point, an esteemed academician took the stage, gestured to Boothman, and indicated that the process would "singlehandedly bankrupt the University of Michigan." The academician's contention was that providing honest communication to patients following an adverse medical event or medical error would expose participating hospitals and through them, the physicians, to a greater number of malpractice suits and huge legal fees that would, in turn, lead to "an insurmountable mountain of debt."

Nor was the esteemed academician the only one to scoff at Boothman's efforts to focus on communication and resolution following the occurance of a medical error. During the mid-2000s, a New York judge was unsympathetic to the concept in the face of medical error, telling Boothman that he was "taking advantage of people in their most vulnerable moment," by offering immediate compensation for less money than they might receive through litigation and trial by jury, even if that litigation might end up in an unfavorable verdict (Smith 2019). Given that medical academicians and legal experts, at the time, believed that physician disclosure of error could cause more harm than positive benefits, we begin to see why it was difficult for physicians to acknowledge wrongdoing when it came to a mistake or failure of treatment.

That a disclosure could either be the cause of, or find its way as evidence into, a lawsuit is one compelling reason why practitioners stay silent. I've already mentioned that litigation takes up large amounts of time and leads to a great deal of expense. Furthermore, according to Sage (2005), physicians regarded malpractice suits as "unjustified affronts to medical professionalism," while Studdert, Mello, and Brennan, in 2004, pointed out that physicians consider malpractice suits as punishment for random events that create unwanted expense and extreme emotional pain. This perceived affront to the physicians is further exacerbated by risk managers and legal counsel telling physicians the (more often than not falsehood) that apologizing for errors will inevitably lead to legal actions on the part of the patient or his or her family. Such fear, to an extent, has been a large obstacle when it comes to implementing and maintaining any kind of disclosure plan (Mello, Armstrong, Greenberg, McCotter, and Gallagher, 2016). In addition, there is also an inherent difficulty when it comes to showing that apologies reduce risk. Asks Welch (2011), "How do you measure lawsuits that do not occur?"

In addition to outright fear, other reasons exist as to why it can be difficult for physicians to apologize for wrongdoing.

### *Discomfort of Acknowledging a Mistake*

I've stated, throughout this book, the obvious fact that no one likes making mistakes. Doing so, and owning up to them, is an uncomfortable process, as it means we aren't infallible and that we are capable of error. It can also mean that we might have unwittingly harmed another individual through that error. This feeling is magnified a great deal among physicians, not only when it comes to making mistakes, but also when it comes to owning up to them.

Many physicians seriously believe they shouldn't be in a position to make mistakes. They are, after all, responsible for the successful treatment of patients. A medical error can negatively affect a patient. As such, it should come as no surprise that when an adverse error takes place under a physician's watch, there is a great deal of shame and guilt that comes along with making that mistake (Leape, 2012; see also Davidoff, 2002). Added to this factor, physicians have very high standards and quite rightly so. They are dedicated to providing the highest-quality care for their patients and do their best to adhere to that ideal. As such, when something goes wrong, and these physicians make mistakes, they believe that they have not only failed the patients but themselves, as well. Basically,

> we are asking physicians to perform an extremely difficult and sensitive human interaction at the time when they feel most vulnerable and inadequate. They need help, and too often, the institution and their colleagues do not provide it. (Leape, 2012)

Not only does a mistake mean the physician has failed a patient. In his or her own eyes, being the cause of a medical error means the physician has failed him- or herself. Within this emotional context, it can be agonizingly difficult for a doctor to admit disclosure or apologize for a mistake.

### Risk Managers

A health-care system's risk management department is in charge of, well, managing risk. That is the nature of this particular department. As such, these employees are responsible for minimizing any potential risk, or fallout, from actions taken by the organization's staff.

As such, Many risk managers subscibe to the idea that apologies in the face of medical error aren't appropriate, nor are they needed, unless a poor outcome was preventable or unless the organization was responsible for the adverse event (Welch, 2011). As a result, a health-care provider and organization might be strongly encouraged not to make an apology, even if it could make the practitioner feel better for unburdening him- or herself.

Nor are risk managers the only cause behind nondisclosure; such an action can also speak to the culture of a health-care organization or hospital when it comes to acknowledging medical errors and apologizing for them, especially if the organization's leaders believe the members didn't do anything wrong, which can be the case. Going back to the story of Beth Daley Ullem and the loss of her newborn son, the institution's belief that sometimes bad things happen in the delivery of health care (especially with births) tends to be more the rule than the exception, when it comes to mistakes and errors. As such, the institutions—and their risk managers—shrug the idea of any apologies away, putting it down to the idea that bad things just happen.

### Systems versus Individuals

When an individual makes a mistake, it's easy for that person to apologize and make whatever compensation is reasonable. However, as mentioned earlier, a physician rarely makes a mistake on his or her own. Rather, that mistake can be part of a system breakdown, with the end result that the individual physician is caught holding the bag when a mistake is made.

In this situation, and in the face of an adverse medical event, the individual physician could likely find him- or herself in the position of not only apologizing for the error itself but also for the systems in place that might have led to that error in the first place, as well as the harm and pain that can sometimes come from that mistake (Leape 2012). As such, a physician could be in the position of making an apology without really knowing what caused the error.

It goes without saying that the consequences of harm or injury from an adverse medical event can sometimes be severe. The consequences of harm or injury can be substantial; the patient could end up with a lifelong disability. The more severe the injury or disability, the more difficult the apology. And if injury takes place as part of medical treatment that is put into place to help the patient, the injury could threaten the trust and relationship between the health-care provider and patient.

### *Lack of Sufficient Skills to Make an Apology*

Making a "good" apology is difficult—more often than not, simply saying, "I'm sorry," doesn't do much. As I'll discuss in this book, apologizing properly requires certain features and steps to be effective. With this in mind, it's safe to say that physicians, more often than not, lack sufficient skills for apologizing—they typically haven't received instruction on apologizing in medical school. By the time they make it to their residency programs, newly minted physicians rarely, if ever, witness a senior physician apologizing. As time goes on, medical students and residents end up ignoring their own ethical quandries to fit in with the culture, as they're afraid that their grades—and ultimate success—could depend on it (Lehman, 2008).

As such, during their years of instruction, physicians don't learn the skills for apologizing or how to cope with the concept of apologies, nor do they have role models or mentors who can help them do so. As a result, "they are being asked to do something that is difficult, and for which they feel unprepared and inexperienced," Leape said. "No wonder they feel uncomfortable."

Sara Peskin, who, in 2018, was a neurology resident at the University of Pennsylvania, pointed out that apologies are difficult for physicians because medical schools teach how to examine and treat rather than to "err and recover." "Nobody stands behind a podium and declares: 'Each of you will make mistakes and some of them will hurt people,'" she said (2018). As such, practitioners are not prepared for dealing with how to react when the inevitable mistakes occur.

### *Lack of an Effective Medical Error Reporting / Apology System*

Many health-care institutions don't have a specific system in place by which they can deal with medical errors and their outcomes, not to mention an apology process that can help deflect the outcomes of some of those errors (Poorolajal, Razaie, and Aghighi, 2015). Systems that are in place—such as the aforementioned "Morbidity and Mortality" conferences—are mostly critical in nature, ones in which blame is assigned, rather than effort put toward trying to figure out why the error occurred in the first place. This returns to a failure of institutions and systems when it comes to apologizing or helping to deal with physician mistakes. Physicians don't know how to apologize for mistakes (nor are they encouraged to do so), and the organizations for which they work don't know how to deal with medical errors, other than to assign blame. And, depite it all, malpractice lawsuits can be the end result of not apologizing.

Additionally, there can be a generational conflict within these institutions as to how to handle medical error. Older providers tend to err on the side of silence, deny-and-defend, as they might not know or understand any other way of dealing with mistakes. Meanwhile, their younger colleagues are more interested in acknowledging wrong up front. As such, "all of these systemic factors become more complex when medical errors occur," Lehman observed.

Finally, the focus is misplaced, even when errors or mistakes are acknowledged. "In response (to an error), we fix technology," wrote Peskin. "We don't talk about the emotional trauma of hurting a patient." Physicians also don't escape unscathed; when they make mistakes that cause harm, they must cope with guilt, self-doubt, and the ever-present fear of litigation.

### ◆ The Impact of "Not Sorry" on Patients

Unlike patients treated by early Greek physicians or those who received treatment from doctors in the eighteenth, nineteenth, and early twentieth centuries, today's patients are active participants in their health-care decisions (Cleopas, Villaveces, et al., 2006). Thanks to the Internet especially, patients have a better idea of what might be wrong and what can go wrong with a given procedure. They are no longer in the dark when it comes to medical or treatment options. Armed with this information, patients are able to intelligently talk with their health-care providers about topics pertaining to their health and well-being.

With this in mind, some experts believe that physicians should disclose both harmful and nonharmful events to patients (Chamberlain, Koniarus, Wu, and Pawlik, 2012). However, one study ended up being lukewarm to the concept. The study examined patient and physician emotions following an error, with some interesting results. Patients reported that, in the wake of learning about the error, they felt sad, anxious, depressed, and traumatized (Gallagher, Waterman, Ebers, Fraser, and Levinson, 2003). These patients also feared additional errors and were frustrated that the original errors could have been prevented. Furthermore, while patients indicated needing emotional support following an error and its disclosure, physicians, in maintaining what they consider an appropriate professional demeaner when discussing the error, are coming across as cold and unfeeling. This study didn't, however, suggest that the patients would immediately go to their phones and call their lawyers because of the adverse events in which they were involved. Nor did it suggest that the patients didn't want the error to be disclosed or that the patient wasn't anticipating some type of apology when it came to the error's disclosure.

Ackerman (2018), in the meantime, discussed a story in the *Washington Post*, involving a study that compared and contrasted medical errors and their disclosures following patients' "devastating consequences during surgery." One patient was faced by a "white wall of silence," in which that individual was told nothing. The other patient received an immediate explanation by and apology from his surgeon. The result of both apology and disclosure led to the patient and physician becoming "engaged in productive discussions with risk managers," with the result being a confidential settlement agreement, without litigation (Ackerman, 2018; see also Boodman, 2017). While this is one scenario in one error situation, it showed that, for the most part, patients want information in the face of an adverse medical event.

Another study found that even in situations in which physicians disclosed information about an adverse event, they avoided indicating that an error occurred, why it occurred, or how similar errors would be prevented in the future. This, in turn, meant that patients were left wanting with the lack of information; they wanted a better understanding about why the error had occurred, what it might mean for their health, how the problem would be corrected, and how future errors might be prevented. One patient, in fact, described the type of full disclosure and apology he would have liked to have received, following an insulin overdose:

> I'm sorry, but due to an error of writing instructions and communications there was a misunderstanding, and it caused an overdose of insulin. You have my deepest sympathy as far as physical problems that we caused for you. However, we're doing everything within our powers to correct this error, and we can assure you that this problem will not happen again. I'm not only going to address it as far as writing the information down, but I'm also going to communicate it, so the nurse will understand what is supposed to be given ... I'm available to sit down and discuss with you, in detail, what happened, and again, I'm sorry.

Aside from the desire simply to know what went wrong, from the patient/family viewpoint, physicians and health-care organizations who treat them and their families as financial threats and liabilities following an adverse medical event leave them feeling abandoned, while ensuring that the health-care system ends up exposing other patients to the same poor health outcome (Boothman, 2016; see also Marcus, 2002). Feelings of betrayal are also common; it's one thing to make a mistake, but simply dismissing the mistake as nothing important can seriously erode the trust a patient has in a physician.

This feeling of abandonment and betrayal, in fact, is one of the main reasons why patients end up seeking legal advice and decide on lawsuits in the wake of a medical error that isn't disclosed. Many aren't interested in compensation; they simply want to know the truth behind a mistake. Such a truth can typically come out during the "discovery" phase of litigation or even during trial.

"Studies suggest that, the majority of lawsuits result from people not being able to get information, and suing out of the sheer desire to know what happened, plus anger, once they've been stonewalled," according to Albert Wu, MD, a Johns Hopkins professor and editor of the *Journal of Patient Safety and Risk Management* (Smith, 2019).

Such anger can also affect patient retention and the physician-patient relationship, not to mention seriously damage public perception of a medical practice or health-care system. This is the case, especially in this day and age of social media, in which Facebook posts and tweets can go viral in a matter of minutes.

To reiterate, silence following an adverse medical event leads a patient to distrust the practitioner or organization that is treating him or her. In the face of such silence and (perceived) indifference, the patient can experience emotions ranging from frustration and anger to depression and betrayal. As the silence continues, and little to no information is forthcoming, the patient may find him- or herself calling a lawyer and filing suit, just to find out the cause of a particular adverse medical event.

## ◆ The Impact of "Not Sorry" on Physicians

A lack of apology following a medical error or adverse event does more than make a patient or family angry or depressed or launch a potential malpractice lawsuit. It can provide emotional harm to the physician, as well.

Helo and Moulton (2017) point out, quite rightly, that physicians, much like pilots, "carry a greater burden, as their errors can be castrophic." If pilots make mistakes, they run the risk of harming the passengers they are entrusted to carry. Physicians, by the same token, can also create harm if they make mistakes; I have reiterated, throughout this book, that medicine is a highly dangerous practice. Physicians don't go into a procedure or prescribe a treatment with the idea that it will fail. So when the said procedure or treatment does fail, it can result in serious harm to a patient (and that patient's family), as well as emotional consequences for the health-care provider. These emotional consequences can become worse, if physicians aren't allowed to apologize or make amends, because the organization in which they are practicing tells them not to do so.

In the aforementioned study by Ackerman concerning patient and physician emotional reactions to medical errors, physicians also experienced powerful emotions following a medical error (Ackerman, 2018). Understandably, they felt upset and guilty about harming the patient, disappointed about feeling like failures and not meeting their own high standards, fearful about a potential lawsuit, and anxious about any repercussions, including the impact on their reputations (Gallagher, Waterman, Ebers, Fraser, and Levinson, 2003).

Part of the reason for this is because physicians are thought (and taught) to be infallable (and the culture in which they operate underlines this fact). This is probably a good thing—you don't want a surgeon operating on you if he or she doubts his or her abilities to do a good job. However, physicians are as human as the patients they treat. This means that they can also experience the same guilt and shame when it comes to making mistakes as the rest of us do.

Helo and Moulton (2017) discuss publications from the mid-1980s that described physicians' guilt, shame, and inadequacy following medical errors. This idea, in turn, led both Wu (2000) and Scott et al. (2009) to name physicians as "second victims" when it comes to an adverse medical event. Such a syndrome means that physicians can suffer as much, if not more, than patients when adverse events take place, and they aren't able to apologize for them.

This is because physicians who make mistakes during procedures, treatment, or care feel personally responsible for the patient outcome, especially if that outcome leads to death or disability. Many feel as though they've failed the patient and furthermore end up second-guessing themselves and their skills and knoweldge base, especially when it comes to future procedures. Wu, a physician himself, delves into a deeper explanation about the impact of a mistake on a physician:

> Virtually every practitioner knows the sickening realization of making a bad mistake. You feel singled out and exposed—seized by the instinct to see if anyone has noticed. You agonise about what to do, whether to tell anyone, what to say. Later, the event

replays itself over and over in your mind. You quesiton your competence but fear being discovered. You know you should confess, but dread the prospect of potential punishment and the patient's anger.

Furthermore, physicians who believe themselves responsible for medical errors undergo six phases of the "second victim" syndrome. These are as follows:

- chaos and accident response
- intrusive reflections
- restoring personal integrity
- enduring the inquisition
- obtaining emotional first aid
- moving on

The problem, however, is that the second victims might not be allowed the steps necessary to restore personal integrity or obtain emotional first aid. Rather than being permitted an outlet available to most of us—an apology—they are, instead, forced to endure either silence or an inquisition, during which they are blamed for committing an error that they are already beating themselves up over. This can make "moving on" very difficult, if not impossible. This has prompted Wu to point out that there is no room for mistakes when it comes to modern medicine, a philosophy that is similar in nature to that outlined in the Code of Hammurabi. While physicians are human beings, everything from technology to lab test prescision to innovations has "created an expectation of perfection," Wu commented. Furthermore, whether they mean to or not, patients collude with doctors to deny the existence of error.

Furthermore, while patients and their families can turn to various sources to deal with the emotional outcomes of an adverse medical event, physicians have few, if any, mechanisms available when they make a mistake. As mentioned earlier, the institutions for which these providers work tend to "circle the wagons" and do what they can to prevent potential litigation. Physicians are told to keep quiet and not talk to the patients or their families or to share what went wrong. This culture of silence means physicians themselves find ways to cope or protect themselves emotionally. They can often lash out with anger, blame others, and even scold the patient or other members of the health-care team. Physicians also cope by "denial, discounting, and distancing." In addition, this distress can escalate during the many years of a malpractice suit, with many burning out, losing their nerve, or escalating drinking or drug use.

There is a reason why Helo and Moulton point out that "mistakes are ubiquitous in medicine, yet providers are often unprepared to deal with the aftermath of a medical error." When a physician makes a mistake, not only is he or she not allowed to directly apologize, but the physician also doesn't have an outlet for the inevitable guilt and shame that comes with making a mistake. This can create more emotional problems for this provider, which could affect this individual's ability to adequately care for future patients.

Leape (2012) is adamant that hospitals and health-care systems should take responsibility for medical errors and implement and support apology training programs. Yet, while many hospitals are initiating such programs, there are reasons why others do not. The main reason is because hospital executives believe it isn't appropriate for them to interfere with a physician and his or her medical practice, a concept that doctors have supported. Additionally, hospital lawyers have typically counseled against full disclosure and apology, believing that going down that path can increase the likelihood of a lawsuit and losing in court.

On the positive side, physicians are slowly leaning toward more disclosure. However, studies have shown a large variation concerning how health-care providers disclose mistakes to patients (Gallagher et al., 2006). For example, Gallagher noted that, of more than 2,500 physicians surveyed in the United States and Canada, 56 percent chose statements that mentioned the adverse event but not the error itself, 42 percent explicitly stated that an error occurred, 19 percent wouldn't volunteer information about the error's cause, and 63 percent wouldn't provide specific information about how future errors might be prevented. Additionally, disclosure was affected by the nature of the error and the health-care specialty.

The takeaways from this particular section are that

1) Medical error occurs, probably more frequently than we are aware of, because health-care providers are human and mistakes happen.
2) Unfortunately, because of the structure of various health-care systems, transparency, acknowledgment, and apologies can be few and far between.
3) Lack of transprency, "deny-and-defend," and other methods of retaining information mean the patient is in the dark about what happened. Physicians are also told to keep quiet.

The wall of silence can lead the patient and his or her family to a lawsuit in an effort to obtain the needed information or to receive some kind of financial compensation for pain or injury.
4) The way in which health-care systems and hospitals are set up doesn't provide for the possibility of medical error, how to deal with it, or how to handle it. As such, there is no effort to ensure that said errors are corrected.
5) A lack of apology can have dire consequences on the patient and family (who feel abandoned and frustrated with the lack of transparency), as well as the physician (who feels guilt, shame, and remorse but doesn't have an outlet to express these feelings).

What I've proved in the preceding section is that silence in the face of medical errors can have dire effects, including emotional issues for both patients and their doctors, leading to litigation.

The next question here is, can a simple apology help reduce litigation and provide closure to the patients/families who were the victims of the errors and the physicians who were responsible for them? The answer to this question is yes—to an extent. Apologizing can be considered a good first step following an adverse medical event. However, it's important that the apology be structured and delivered in a way in which patients (and their families) are satisfied and physicians receive some sort of absolution. In other words, a simple "I'm sorry" won't necessary solve the issue. What needs to happen involves everything from training to a revamped organizational structure, which I'll explore in the next sections.

# ANATOMY OF AN APOLOGY

THE PREVIOUS SECTIONS DELVED DEEPLY INTO A HIStory of medical error, the need for disclosure of such error, and why divulging and apologizing for making a mistake is more the exception than the norm in a health-care situation. As mentioned before, dealing with an adverse medical event requires more than a simple "I'm sorry." In fact, in examining the anatomy of an apology, we find that an effective one should focus on more than a verbal expression of remorse. In this section, I'll examine what, exactly, an apology consists of, and then focus on the ways in which these apologies can, and should, be used as a response to medical error and avoiding potential litigation.

◆ **Definition**

In their most basic sense, apologies are "an acknowledgment of harm and admission of responsibility" (Okimoto, Wenzel, and Hedrick, 2013). In such a situation, apologies are often considered to be what Okimoto et al. (2013) dub an "equity-restoring response," one in which "offenders remove power from their victims" in a symbolic sense. What happens in an apology is that a perpetrator apologizes for committing a wrong, the victim who has been wronged accepts and forgives the perpetrator, and both can move on.

Winch (2010) points out that most people believe that an apology should include three basic ingredients: 1) a statement of regret for what happened, 2) a clear "I'm sorry" statement, and 3) a request for forgiveness. But Winch goes further, suggesting that a true apology needs other ingredients:

- expression of empathy
- offer of compensation
- acknowledgment that certain rules or norms were violated

Winch also reminds us that apologies are going to differ, based on the relationships and situations in question. Specifically, an apology to a spouse for forgetting an anniversary will differ from an apology to a work colleague for forgetting a contribution to another coworker's birthday party. In such cases, when apologizing to a spouse, the empathy component should be the focus. The co-worker apology, in the meantime, should have a more specific focus on the offer of compensation.

Moving on to the field of medicine, Lazare, in 2004, pointed out that, when it comes to patients who have been wronged, apologies can be therapeutic in the following ways:

- An apology restores the patient's dignity and self-respect.
- An apology offers assurances of shared values between physician / health-care provider and the patient.

- An apology assures a patient that he or she is not at fault. Self-blame tends to be a common patient response to injury, something that physicians might not be aware of (see also Leape, 2012). To reiterate, patients often know when something has gone wrong, though they can't always put their finger on what that "wrong" might be.
- An apology assures the patient that he or she is safe when it comes to care and treatment and that the health-care provider is taking every step possible to prevent additional or further injury.
- An apology also shows the patient that the doctor is suffering, thus leveling the playing field and helping to restore that patient's self-respect. The apology also allows the patient to forgive the doctor.
- An apology demonstrates that the health-care provider and the institution backing him or her understand the victim's suffering and loss of trust, especially if the particular apology involves making amends or offering compensation.

Additionally, the end benefit of an apology should include the following:

- diffusing an otherwise complex situation
- negating emotion, neutralizing communication
- downgrading potential anger associated with the occurrence
- providing respect toward the patient or patient's family

## ◆ Benefits of Apologizing

The proper use of apologizing for just about anything, including adverse medical events, can provide a great many benefits.

Allan and McKillop (2010) present the idea that a patient or patient's family who might have been wronged wants to forgive and that forgiveness can help reduce negative physical reactions to an adverse event. If the physician who made the mistake apologizes, it allows the patient and his or her family to forgive, and this can go a long way toward helping the physician to heal from his or her mistake and to forgive him- or herself as well for making that mistake.

This idea that apologies can have positive physical ramifications is supported by actual research; Allan and McKillop note that decreased immunity, combined with digestive problems and release of stress hormones, tends to be the result of the stress of unforgiveness, which happens when no apology or expression of remorse is forthcoming from the perpetrator. That stress, in turn, can impair any kind of health recovery (see also Worthingon and Scherer, 2004). Instead, the lack of honesty or apology can create anxiety within a patient, which, in turn, could lead to a release of certain hormones that might prevent any kind of healing.

It doesn't take research to understand this; anyone who is under stress knows the physical symptoms—the shortness of breath, digestive issues, headaches, and other manifestations. While the psychological response of stress focuses on "cognitive, affective and behavioral facets," the physiological reaction involves a higher blood pressure rate and perspiration, as the body's autonomic nervous system and hypothalamus, pituitary gland, and adrenal cortex are activated (Allan and McKillop, 2010; see also Worthington and Scherer, 2004). In other words, individuals confronted with an adverse medical event are likely to become stressed, which can evidence itself in the form of higher blood pressure and heart rate. In other words, patients can suffer twice—first, as victims of doctor error and second, as the stress created by a wall of silence triggers physical responses, making the situation that much more untenable and leading to that infamous legal statement of "pain and suffering."

The key to forgiveness, Allan and McKillop note, can be a well-crafted apology. And that apology needs to be more than an expression of regret following an adverse event. Allan and McKillop point out that a full apology—one that is likely to acknowledge the occurrence of an adverse event and help reduce the physiological effects—consists of an admission of responsibility for causing the harm, an expression of regret, some kind of action to remedy the harm of what's been done, and an explanation of how future occurences will be prevented from happening (see also Robbennolt, 2003, and Alan, 2008).

An expression of regret and error disclosure, in fact, can help patients develop a more positive perception of the health-care providers in question who might have perpetrated the event. Certainly, the patients and their families might still blame the professionals for the adverse event. However, in the face of a sincere expression of remorse and offer of compensation, the intensity of that blame should be reduced. Boiling this down, the concept of "honesty is the best policy," in this case, has a measure of truth to it.

Another benefit is that when a physician apologizes, patients are considered better able to develop empathy with the professionals. Empathetic patients, especially, understand that unintended outcomes do occur, that to err is human, that other circumstances might have contributed to the incident in question, and that they themselves might also be to blame for any potential adverse event. Specifically, just about everyone accepts the fact that human beings make mistakes, and that's fine. Basically, this expression of remorse makes doctors more human and less cold or institutional.

Furthermore, patients who are the victims of adverse events often want assurances and actions taken so that the harm will be corrected, that their immediate needs will be taken care of, and that a repeat of similar events in the future won't take place, either with their own care or that of other patients (see also Ledema et al., 2008). As such, a sincere expression of regret (with emphasis on the "sincere") can work toward ensuring that a patient's physiological issues can be lessened through the ability to forgive. Furthermore, patients can experience a sense of relief from such an apology.

Yet, it isn't only patients who receive benefits from a correctly delivered apology. Leape (2012) and others also point out that healthcare providers and doctors who err also need healing. I explained in the preceding section that physicians can be the "second victims" of error nondisclosure, and sitting on an apology because of advice not to apologize can create more harm than good. Apologizing provides that first step in healing, offering the physician a method by which he or she can deal with the normal shame and guilt of making a mistake. Through such an apology, the physician is asking those he or she has wronged for forgiveness. As mentioned earlier, the patient and families want to grant that forgiveness and are ready to do so in the face of the physician's expression of remorse. Once forgiveness is received, both parties can move on. But without the apology mechanism in place, a patient is stuck in limbo, not wanting to forgive, while a physician isn't able to receive that forgiveness. In such a situation, moving on can be highly difficult, if not impossible.

### ◆ The Art of Apologizing

A very good example of the use of apologizing to acknowledge harm and to take responsibility can be found in the Jewish religion, which follows the Hebrew, or lunar, calendar. To Jews, two of the most important holidays take place in the fall: Rosh Hashanah (known as the Jewish New Year) and Yom Kippur, the Day of Atonement. The new year offers celebration and renewal—it's called the "Birthday of the World" for many reasons.

On the day of Yom Kippur, observant Jews will spend most of their time in prayer, beseeching God to forgive them for their transgressions and allowing them to wipe the slate clean. These two events are known as the "High Holidays." And the ten days taking place between these two holidays are known as the "Days of Awe." During such time, Jews are required to approach those they have wronged during the year, even unknowingly, and to apologize for that wrongdoing. The idea here is that the Days of Awe allow those who are repentant for what they've done to clean their emotional slate and start fresh in the New Year.

While the concept of "apologizing" is fairly straightforward, Jewish literature is filled with right and wrong ways to apologize to someone who is wronged. And much of that literature is in agreement that simply saying, "I'm sorry," doesn't go far enough.

Heshy Friedman underlines this concept in a somewhat humorous fashion, presenting what he calls "arguably the worst apology ever." The "worst apology" comes from a clip of the classic television show *The Honeymooners*, during which Ralph Kramden attempts to record an apology to his wife, Alice, for calling her mother a blabbermouth (Friedman, 2012; see also Russel and Finn, 1956):

> Hello, Alice. This is me, Ralph. Alice, I'm sorry. I'm miserable without you. Please come back to me, Alice. I apologize for everything I said. I even apologize to your mother. I know she doesn't mean the things she says, Alice. It's just her nature. She doesn't mean to be mean. She's just born that way. When she says things about your old boyfriends and about the furniture in the apartment, I know that she doesn't mean to get me mad. She's just naturally mean, that's all. When she spilled the beans about the end of the play, I shouldn't have got mad at that. I should've expected it from her. I know how she is. She's never gonna be any different, Alice! She's gonna be the same old way, Alice! SHE'S A BLABBERMOUTH, ALICE! A BLABBERMOUTH!

"Before apologizing," Friedman suggested, "it might be a good idea to view this video clip, so that you know what not to do."

On a more serious note, Judaism has made apologizing a fine art during the Days of Awe. The Jewish scholar, rabbi, philosopher, and yes, physician Maimonides noted that the four steps toward a proper apology include the following (Harchol and Kaye):

1) verbally confessing the mistake and asking for forgiveness
2) expressing sincere remorse and resolving/promising not to make the same mistake again
3) doing everything to right the wrong and to appease the individual who might have been hurt or wounded
4) acting differently if the situation should happen again

Following these four steps isn't necessarily easy; it isn't meant to be. However, according to Jewish tradition, the steps are necessary to repair the wrong—it falls under the Hebrew concept of *teshuva*, which is important during the ten days linking the Jewish New Year and Day of Atonement (Harchol and Kaye).

The preceding isn't to suggest that other religions don't have their methods of sincere apology. But examination of the apology "how-tos" during the High Holidays is a good way to launch into a discussion about the actual science of apologizing to others for mistakes made. My contention here is that "sorry" isn't enough. Basically, the methods introduced by Maimonides and others represent a good bedrock for today's apology methods from the doctor to the patient and the patient's family, following an adverse medical event. Just as important to realize is that the term *apology* encompasses a wide range of actions. Specifically, not all apologies are created equal.

### ◆ Types of Apologies

Schoenewolf, in 2015, laid out six different apologies, their meanings, and their contexts.

## 1) *Apologizing to appease*

People will often apologize in an attempt to control someone's feelings. For example, if an alcoholic goes on a drinking binge and comes home to his angry wife, he'll apologize in the hope that he can deflect her anger. In this case, the man doesn't truly feel sorry or remorse for what he's done, but he wants to prevent her from getting mad, resulting in more trouble for himself. When it comes to medical error disclosure, such an apology might be made, on the fly, to prevent a patient or patient's family from getting angry at a situation, but there is little true remorse or desire to change / correct the situation that has taken place. There are several things wrong with this type of apology, not the least of which is that it can come across as unfeeling or uncaring, with no real thought or action behind it. What this type of apology suggests is that the doctor is mouthing accepted words to get the patient—and his or her family—off his or her back in the face of an adverse medical event.

## 2) *Apologizing on demand*

Schoenewolf calls this "one of the most common types of apology." We see it all the time in news stories, typically among celebrities or famous athletes who have made mistakes of which the public has become aware. The person in question writes an objectionable or racist comment on Facebook or Twitter, that celebrity's followers/media/the general public become outraged in response, and the person in question backpedals with an apology, which is done out of expediency. Nine times out of ten, such an apology is penned by that person's publicist and read by the offender by rote. There is no true meaning behind the apology. The issue with such apologies, however, is that the person hasn't been punished for his or her crime or comment. This is also the type of apology that might be issued if someone gets caught doing something he or she shouldn't have—that person is not necessarily apologizing for his or her actions. Rather, he or she is responding to being called out in a negative situation.

When it comes to medicine, an example of an apology on demand might be if a physician commits some kind of error, is caught doing so, and apologizes by rote, because the patient or his or her family has created an uproar with the hospital board or even friends and neighbors. Perhaps the physician's risk management department or legal counsel has told him or her to apologize. The physician might do so, but there is no real force behind the apology. The physician got caught making a mistake and is doing what he or she is told by someone else, in an effort to prevent anger, backlash, or a lawsuit. This is not a sincere apology. Similar to the apology to appease, the action suggests little more than words.

**3) *Apologizing without apologizing***

This isn't an apology at all but has the appearances of an apology. Certainly, there is an "I'm sorry" factor with this, but this type of apology takes the form of "I'm sorry if I hurt you," which translated means "I don't think I really did anything to hurt or harm you, but I'm dutifully apologizing in case you think I did." This type of apology (or nonapology, as the case might be) is also used to deflect the wrongdoing ("I'm sorry if you are offended, or feel hurt, by what I did"). It acknowledges potential harm or wrongdoing, but the individual issuing this statement doesn't believe he or she is in the wrong or to blame for the wrongdoing, but rather, it is the victim's perceived feelings that are to blame for feeling bad.

When it comes to medical error, an example of a physician who apologizes without apologizing might be "I'm sorry if this procedure didn't work as planned." This is not an apology. It is deflecting blame to the procedure from the individual in charge of the procedure. In this case, the physician is saying he or she is sorry but isn't really accepting the blame for wrongdoing, nor does it indicate that he or she will change in any way or look into why "the procedure" didn't work. This is not to suggest that the procedure itself never goes awry. However, with this type of apology, there is no culpability or remorse, which is something that the savvy patient will be able to realize.

### 4) *Apologizing out of politeness*

There are people who apologize for every little thing, even if it isn't their fault. If this individual bumps into someone by mistake, he or she issues an automatic apology. Schoenewolf points out that, in this group, people apologize as a way to either show courtesy or to show others how nice and polite they are. "If they graze past somebody in a hallway, they immediately say 'sorry,'" he noted (2015). The phlebotomist who has to draw blood from a patient and says, "I'm sorry if this hurts," isn't really sorry (unless the individual apologizes with empathy, more on that follows). What he or she is indicating is that he or she is being polite and is trying to show the person how nice he or she is by issuing an apology, even though he or she doesn't really mean it. The nurse who accidentally jostles a patient's arm when taking his or her blood pressure and says, "I'm sorry," is also doing so to be polite. This type of apology is one in which the apologizer wants to gain approval or to avoid conflict. What it is saying is "I'm a nice person, and really, I am not a threat to anyone around here." This could be considered a *nonspecific* apology, in that it doesn't really accept or deny blame. Rather, it is apologizing for the sake of apologizing for the sake of being polite.

### 5) *Apologizing with love/empathy*

Schoenewolf calls this "the consummate apology." It is an apology that is made when people truly love and care about someone else. The person making the apology is able to empathize with the pain being experienced by the other person and has a definite sense as to how that other individual might feel. The person delivering the apology wants the other person to know that he or she cares. Though Schoenewolf doesn't say so, this type of apology also implies that steps will be taken to ensure that the situation doesn't repeat itself. By ensuring that the situation doesn't repeat itself, the person apologizing assures the person receiving the apology that similar pain won't be felt by another individual.

This type of apology is the best type, as it not only is an empathetic one, but it also assumes liability. It allows the person who has perpetrated the wrong to basically say, "I messed up. This is why and how I did so, and this is how I will make sure it doesn't happen again in the future." Finally, it also outlines how it will make things right for the person who has been wronged. For example, a physician who is making such an apology might say, "Our fund will pay you a certain amount of money. I know it can't take away the pain of your loss, but I'm hoping this will, at least, help mitigate some of the problem and issue." In short, apologizing with love and empathy allows the physician to show remorse for what happened, allows him or her to own up to the mistake that was committed, and lets him or her explain how that mistake won't happen again and how he or she plans to work with the patient and his or her family to fix the error.

It goes without saying that this is actually the type of apology that should be issued; it provides information to people who have been wronged; it tells them why the situation happened; it provides transparency, remorse, and compensation—all this can help avoid litigation. Perhaps unsurprisingly, however, most health-care organizations don't train their health-care providers as to how to apologize with love or empathy. The end result is an opaque wall when it comes to the "why" of an error. If that wall remains opaque and no one is willing to acknowledge wrongdoing, then that could ultimately lead to litigation.

### ◆ A Reluctance to Own Up

But if apologizing for adverse medical events presents so many benefits and can help defer litigation, why are health-care providers, physicians, health-care systems, and hospitals so reluctant to do so? I mentioned earlier several institutional reasons why an apology for wrongdoing might not be forthcoming; among the top reasons is the admission of wrongdoing might lead to a lawsuit or some other kind of legal action. But research is also showing that, at times, a refusal to apologize might have ramifications other than those of the legal type.

For one thing, Okimoto et al. (2013) notes that an apology can function as a form of self-censure on the part of the person making the apology, in other words, the individual who made the mistake or error in the first place. An apology that refuses to admit any kind of wrongdoing (such as a polite apology or an on-demand apology) can also mean that the wrongdoer's consistency and idealized self-concept remains intact (Okimoto, et al., 2013). In other words, the individual feels that if he or she says he or she is sorry (through, for example, an apology to appease) this, in turn, can reduce "self-oriented dissonance," while maintaining the sense of self-integrity. The individual making a mistake and issuing a non-meaningful apology ensures that his or her ego isn't harmed.

The belief here is that the individual tells him- or herself he or she has said "sorry," that should be enough, and it's time to move on. In contrast, apologizing with empathy, showing remorse, and taking blame for an adverse event can erode an individual's sense of self, which can, in turn, lead to a negative dissonance.

Such negative dissonance can be common in the medical field, in which physicians literally have the power of life and death over their patients. Over time, physicians truly believe they are givers and supporters of life and that their work and efforts are infallable and should not be subject to mistakes or errors. Armed with this belief, some physicians truly believe that accidents or injuries happening to patients are the fault of others, such as the nurse who inadvertently gave the wrong type of medicine because she couldn't read the doctor's instructions or the med tech who was unable to find a vein from which to draw blood for testing. Forcing a physician with this self- and worldview to apologize without appropriate training or understanding can create more problems than it might solve, simply because this individual genuniely believes he or she can do no wrong and hasn't done anything wrong in the case of an adverse medical event.

Beth Daley Ullem ran into this when she lost her newborn son through medical error. As mentioned in the first paragraph of this book, Daley Ullem received no apology or remorse from the hospital in question. Rather, the chief of obstetrics and gynecology—the man who headed up the department and should have taken responsibility for the issue—told her, "You know, sometimes bad things happen. We don't know why God needed your angel, but now you have an angel" (Smith, 2019).

Certainly, this is a terrible thing to say to a grieving mother who only wants answers as to what happened (and who ended up suing the doctors and hospital simply to obtain that information). This situation is also a very good example of the dissonance to which Okimo et al. referrred. The mistake wasn't anyone's fault. It was clearly "God's will," and from the perspective of the obstectrics and gynecology chief, that was a good enough explanation. None of the doctors, nurses, or other providers did anything wrong.

Looking at this another way, admission of wrongdoing in the death of this newborn would create a huge dissonance in the physician's self-worth and ego, not to mention the self-worth of the department and hospital that employs the physician. Obtaining an apology from such a person or institution will be difficult to impossible, as the wrongdoer would likely believe he is infallable and didn't commit any mistakes—it was, after all, divine province that took the little baby. As a result, the physician is only paying lip service to the action and isn't showing remorse or any indication that the offending behavior is being corrected. This was actually the case with Daley Ullem; the hospital, as mentioned, had a history of similar events, and when Daley Ullem sued, they actually attempted to destroy records of her birth. Deflection aside, this is not the type of institution that is going to issue an appropriate apology that might stave off a lawsuit.

As such, just insisting that a health-care provider apologize for wrongdoing even if a hospital wants to go that far (which, in many situations, simply isn't the case) isn't going to do the trick. Training that focuses on the dissonance of a heartfelt apology and that takes into account the feeling of the person who is responding to the wrongdoing needs to be in place. Otherwise, an apology and acknowledgment of error isn't going to do much good for either the institution or the patient or family who believe they've been wronged.

Along these lines, it's also possible that, in such a situation, the actual wrongdoer should be kept away from making the apology. Rather, a representative of the institution, one who is trained in proper apology protocol, should be offered up to make the apology, show remorse, and promise that the cause of the error will be investigated and the same thing will not happen again.

To conclude this discussion, "I'm sorry" is a nice thought, but issuing these words will likely not get a patient to back down from a lawsuit or help resolve an issue. As we saw earlier, there are many different types of apologies and not all of them are effective. Furthermore, Richard Boothman, one of the early pioneers of the CRP movement, indicated that while basic apologies can, and do, save money and mitigate some of the issues coming from an adverse medical event, "highlighting the role of an apology (can represent) little more than a claims management tactic ... (which serves) to undervalue ... the pivotal role honesty plays in patient safety, functionality and culturally" (Boothman, Imhoff, and Campbell Jr., 2012). In discussing the University of Michigan Health System's model of transparency (see more later in this book), Boothman et al. pointed out that the entire claims management process is just one part of a culture shift that requires a focus on patient safety. Claims considerations, in this light, end up in the background. In other words, without an organizational culture shift and appropriate training, an apology is just an empty effort, one that might not do much to avoid malpractice litigation.

### ◆ Apology Laws—Do They Work?

As many physicians and health-care institutions didn't want to apologize for wrongdoing on their own, even after *To Err Is Human* was released, politicians stepped in to force them to do so. While the Clinton-Obama-backed National Medical Error Disclosure and Compensation Bill (which included the creation of a federal apology law) didn't make it to the floor for a vote, that issue didn't deter states from passing their own apology laws in an attempt to get health-care institutions to apologize for making mistakes. It was felt that if the act of apology was legislated, that such actions could lead to a reduction in lawsuits.

Between 1999 and 2011, the number of states with apology laws increased from two to 38 (McMichael, Van Horn, and Viscusi, 2019). These laws were put into place as part of a tort reform. The reasoning here was that if health-care providers were required, by law, to apologize for adverse medical events, patients would be less likely to sue. This, in turn, would mean fewer resources being spent on malpractice lawsuits. This, at least, is the theory.

In 2002, Pennsylvania became the first state to introduce a legal duty on hospitals to notify a patient or his or her family of an adverse event in writing, within seven days of the event (Liebman and Hyman, 2004). The "serious event," according to the law, is defined as "an event, occurrence or situation involving the clinical care of a patient in a medical facility that resuslts in death or compromises patient safety, and results in an unanticipated injury requiring the delivery of additional health care services to the patient" (Liebman and Hyman, 2004).

Nevada and Florida followed, and the mandatory disclosure laws boosted disclosure efforts from the Joint Commission on Accreditation of Healthcare Organizations, the American Medical Association's Council on Ethical and Judicial Affairs, and the *American College of Physicians Ethics Manual*. Despite those ethical standards, however, physicians continue resisting disclosure of serious adverse events. Part of this is because the nature of apology laws focuses on avoiding malpractice, which certainly is important. But it can still leave a patient wanting.

Apology laws are an important factor when it comes to debate over medical malpractice liability, litigation reduction, and tort reform (McMichael, 2019). As mentioned earlier, one reason why defendants, especially those in the health-care arena, have been dissuaded against apologizing is because apologies themselves could be considered evidence of wrongdoing, which, in turn, could increase the likelihood that victims might seek out redress through legal means. Apologies could also be offered into evidence in the event that a malpractice suit makes it all the way to a trial by jury. The idea here is that if an apology, by law, can't be used as evidence or to spark a lawsuit, it will mean that the practitioner will be more willing to apologize for wrongdoing. Specifically, depending on the state in which they were issued, apology laws attempt to help the facilitation of physicians' admission of wrongdoing by reducing or eliminating the risk connected with apologies for adverse medical events.

The question here becomes whether legislating apologies actually has an impact on aggrieved patients filing lawsuits or lessens the chances of such a lawsuit being started in the first place. Benjamin McMichael, assistant professor of law at the University of Alabama School of Law, believes that apology legislation doesn't work—he has, in fact, written several research papers on the topic supporting his stance.

He defines apology law as "reforms to state evidentiary codes that prohibit a plaintiff from introducing into evidence a statement of apology, sympathy or condolence by the defendant" (McMichael, 2018, 1201; see also Ho and Liu, 2011). The theory in this instance is that once the defendant no longer fears having an apology introduced as evidence in a litigation situation, he or she is in a better position to apologize to the plaintiff. In such a situation (again, in theory), the defendant can benefit from the apology, while avoiding the costs.

But McMichael explains that apology laws are in place more as tort reforms, as opposed to any kind of formal changes to state rules of evidence. To that end, the goal of apology laws is to reduce the risk of a lawsuit being filed while encouraging a quick resolution of suits that are filed. He also noted that "apology laws now outstrip more familiar tort reforms, such as noneconomic damages caps in popularity among states."

There are a couple of reasons for the failure of apology legislation, one of which is that apology laws are specifically directed toward medical malpractice, with the bulk of those laws focused mostly on actions against health-care providers. As such, McMichael et al. points out that apology laws have failed as tort reforms and, in fact, have increased the practice of defensive medicine or overuse of diagnostic testing in an effort to avoid malpractice litigation. Why is this the case?

One reason goes back to the idea of the definition of a "correct" apology. McMichael contends that current apology laws in existence force physicians and health-care providers to deliver ineffective apologies, which, in turn, "signal the occurrence of malpractice to patients who otherwise would not have discovered it." In other words, forcing a physician to apologize for wrongdoing by making it the law to do so could end up with more repercussions than saying nothing at all. Patients are smart enough to realize the difference between a sham apology and one that is sincere. This, in turn, means the physician's risk of malpractice claims increases in the face of a "mandated" apology and, as a result, an increased practice of defensive medicine and higher health-care costs.

Another reason for the failure of apology laws to create fewer lawsuits is based in the reason why victims and families of adverse medical events file lawsuits in the first place. The filing isn't so much based on wanting to receive compensation or a huge payout, as much as it is to acquire the necessary information as to why an adverse event took place, as well as assurance that such an event won't take place again. Apology laws require medical practitioners to apologize; they don't specify that the practitioner needs to explain the reason why a bad situation took place. Furthermore, because these "mandated" apologies don't require a level of detail, they can show up as an insincere effort to make things right. Again, an effective apology is one in which the person apologizing owns up to the wrongdoing, shows remorse, and then demonstrates willingness to change the behavior so the situation won't happen again. Mandating "sorry" doesn't do any of that.

Additionally, states have enacted apology laws in an attempt to avoid malpractice suits while limiting the severity of those that are filed. The problem, however, is that not all apology laws are created equal (much as not all apologies are created equal). Laws can be categorized as either "partial apology laws" or "full apology laws." The partial apology laws protect statements of sympathy or apology but don't protect a health-care provider from making a statement admitting fault, error, or negligence (McMichael, 2018; see also Ho and Liu, 2011).

Meanwhile, the "full apology law" protects all statements, including those of admitted wrongdoing, while protecting additional statements of fault, error, or liability. Basically, depending on which state the physician operates in, he or she might still have concerns about making an apology, even under the law, out of fear he or she might not be protected from a lawsuit.

Furthermore, an apology law can cheapen the meaning or action of an apology. This is because the wrongdoer, in this case, doesn't have anything to lose by apologizing. In fact, the wrongdoer is required, by law, to apologize. It's easy to say "I'm sorry" and not mean it. And when it comes to apology laws, apologies can be used as a strategic tool to reduce legal risk and to get the patient and his or her family off the physician's figurative neck. What the apology law is not is an actual tool to create meaningful reform in the health-care system or to offer the patient or patient's family information.

With this in mind, it should come as no surprise that there is a contrast between proper apologies issued from a health-care organization and its physicians because it's the right thing to do and apologies issued from that same organization because it is a legal requirement. The former focuses on some kind of training in the art of meaningful apologies or disclosure. Specifically, physicians in hospital apology programs are typically trained in when to apologize and what to say as part of a specific disclosure system. Apology laws, in contrast, do not offer any kind of "how-to" training guide, meaning the physician, at best, might not offer the proper apology, which could, at worst, lead to a lawsuit. Again, that physician is going through the motions without showing any real remorse for wrongdoing or making suggestions that could lead to any kind of meaningful organizational change. In addition, apology laws leave out the fact that the physician needs an emotional support network when it comes to mistakes.

In addition, apology laws might suffer from what McMichael et al. (2019) calls "poor statutory design." Similar to most legislation, apology laws are likely the result of legislative compromise and "horse trading." This can mean such laws don't protect, or allow, the type of information necessary for such apologies to prevent patients from filing suit in the face of an adverse event or wrongdoing (McMichael, 2018; see also Mastroianni, Mello, Sommer, Hardy, and Gallagher, 2010). What this is saying is that even if the physician obeys the law and apologizes, the patient could go ahead and file a lawsuit anyway.

Let's look at an example. If the particular apology law in question protects only a physician's statement of sympathy (while not protecting information as to why a particular adverse event took place), that physician might not be able to fully explain the nature of a particular mistake or even how a change might occur to ensure such an event won't take place again. In fact, the physician might be told by his or her risk-management department not to disclose anything of the type. However, this is information a patient wants to have and needs. As such, with only the apology action protected and without the information as to why an adverse event took place, the result could be an increase, rather than decrease, in a patient's feelings of betrayal or anger at the adverse event and its outcome.

In addition, even if the patient or family's anger decreases following an apology, that patient might be prompted to search for information that isn't forthcoming (as it isn't protected under the apology laws). This, in turn, hides the information behind a veil of secrecy. The patient and his or her family, in an effort to find that information, might turn to the legal system as a result and for recourse.

As such, the limited protection offered by apology laws could actually encourage, rather than discourage, malpractice claims and lawsuits, because patients can't obtain the facts they want from partial apologies or half-hearted attempts to express sympathy in the face of medical mistakes. Furthermore, the results of studies pertaining to apology laws have led researchers and scholars to believe that, as well-meaning as they are meant to be, this type of legislation is highly flawed and doesn't achieve the goal of reducing medical malpractice or liability risk.

This doesn't mean, however, that apology laws should be repealed or jettisoned. They just need to be modified, so that they create positive results. McMichael (2018) points out that these laws could be more effective if "state lawmakers ... turn to more traditional, hospital-specific apology programs that provide physicians with training regarding the effective utilization of apologies." Such programs, when set up correctly, offer specific methods toward successful apologies. The author also noted that such programs can reduce both the instances and severity of malpractice claims. With this in mind, legislation might be better off providing incentives to hospitals and health-care organizations to adopt apology and CRP programs or even to make funds available to initiate and maintain the programs, rather than simply legislating "I'm sorry."

In what might seem to be contrary advice, McMichael suggests that defense attorneys representing physicians should advise their clients *not* to apologize for wrongdoing. This is somewhat an interesting commentary, given the idea that apologies and apology laws are in place to help mollify patients and (hopefully) prevent lawsuits. But as has been mentioned before, physicians untrained in the art of a proper apology can be more dangerous than those who say nothing at all. McMichael's suggestion is that attorneys representing patients should be more willing to investigate potential malpractice if an apology is offered, along with the necessary information that a patient or patient family needs when it comes to the cause of an adverse medical event. Only in that situation can plaintiffs, or claimants, experience some kind of closure. When the victims of adverse medical events have this type of information (along with a well-delivered apology), it can potentially reduce litigation costs or the length of a suit.

To reiterate, while well-meaning, legislating apologies isn't too effective when it comes to reducing litigation. Furthermore, it seems be failing miserably as a key to tort reform, namely because it is forcing insincerity and is, once again, stoking fear. Again, what is necessary is for organizations to be trained in the art of apologizing.

# THE FAILURE OF MALPRACTICE LITIGATION

IT WAS INDICATED EARLIER IN THIS BOOK THAT PATIENTS and their families often feel shut out in the aftermath of a medical error. If patients and families continue to be shut out, they might turn to the legal system to get the information they need, in an effort to understand why a mistake was made. However, in most cases, a lawsuit is not necessarily the answer and should be avoided. But right now, most patients who believe they have been wronged feel that suing is the only way to get any satisfaction.

The United States is, it seems, a highly litigious society, especially when it comes to suing doctors for poor treatment, both perceived and actual. According to various AMA research reports, more than one in three physicians (34 percent) have had some kind of medical liability lawsuit filed against them at some point in their careers (O'Reilly, 2018). Malpractice is unfortunately considered a cost of doing business in the medical field, but it doesn't necessarily have to be that way.

In examining a standard deny-and-defend approach when it comes to resolving adverse medical events, the path can be predictable:

- A mistake is made, with a patient being injured or dying.
- No information is forthcoming about why the error took place or who is responsible. No apology is forthcoming either. This is not therapeutic or preferable to the patient, who is not feeling his or her best to begin with.
- The patient or patient's family is continually stonewalled when it comes to obtaining information and told mostly that "things happen" or that the mistake wasn't the fault of the practioner. The result is more stress on top of an already stressful situation. The result could also lead to more physical problems for the patient.
- Meanwhile, the health-care provider, who is already feeling guilty and ashamed for having caused the error, might want to apologize and explain but is cautioned against doing so from either legal counsel or risk management.
- In the face of continued silence, and out of frustration, the patient or patient's family sues the physician or health-care system that perpetrated the error.
- Litigation drags on for years, meaning mounting legal costs and ongoing frustration for all parties involved.
- During the process, information about the situation might come out. Then again, it might not. At some point, a settlement offer might be made. If the patient or family feels as though information is forthcoming as well, then the offer might be accepted. If not, then the litigation will continue.
- If the issue reaches trial, the plaintiff needs to relive the whole experience once again, while the practitioner must defend him- or herself from the mistake in front of a jury. Whether

the jury decides in favor of the plaintiff or defendant, both parties are exhausted. If the case is decided in favor of the plaintiff, the physician's reputation could be ruined. If the case is decided in favor of the defendant, the plaintiff is faced with paying court costs and ongoing legal fees. Furthermore, regardless of the result of the trial, the likelihood is that no apology will be forthcoming, and the hospital or system will continue using the same techniques that caused the initial error in the first place.

Adding more insult to a plaintiff's lawsuit, AMA research noted that, "in the vast majority of claims, the plaintiffs do not prevail" (O'Reilly, 2018). While 68 percent of closed claims were either dropped, dismissed, or withdrawn in 2015, the claims imposed more than $30,000 in defense costs. However, of the 7 percent of medical liability claims determined by a trial verdict, 88 percent of those were won by the defendants. Litigation is no way to respond to an adverse medical event. Lawsuits place a burden on the nation's health system, costing tens of billions of dollars each year. AMA president David O. Barbe, MD, said, "Even though the vast majority of claims are dropped, dismissed or withdrawn, the heavy cost associated with a litigious climate takes a significant financial toll on our health care system when the nation is working to reduce unnecessary health care costs." That doesn't say anything about engendering a patient's trust in a health-care situation.

Michael McCoy, a physician who chaired a tort reform task force in Iowa, agrees with the preceding assessment, pointing out the costs of defending malpractice claims—in addition to the "enormous economic and emotional toll on the patients and physicians," such cases can drag on for years (Smith, 2019). And while patients might win the day in court with a hefty compensation payout, this isn't necessarily why patients decide to sue. Yes, there will be those who call their lawyers with the idea that they'll win millions if a case goes to trial. But patients, for the most part, use the law as a way to break the silence surrounding medical errors and to find out why a situation happened. The issue, however, is that using legal means to reach a goal (that goal being the issuance of necessary information, as well as the remote possibility of compensation) ends up costing the plaintiff time, money, and emotional frustration and stress. Certainly, litigation keeps attorneys in business, but it doesn't do much to resolve the issue that prompted a patient to bring suit in the first place.

And while malpractice and tort reform laws are geared to help reduce the number of medical lawsuits filed, they still don't do much to help injured patients (or their families) obtain what research suggests they desire. Again, in the face of an adverse medical event, the patient needs and wants

1) an account of why the harm ocurred,
2) an apology from the health-care professionals involved,
3) information about how similar harms can be avoided in the future, and
4) appropriate restitution for avoidable harm.

It goes without saying that society doesn't want a medical system in which defensive medicine is practiced. It also goes without saying that, despite some stereotypes of trigger-happy patients who want to do nothing more than sue doctors, most patients and their families are not eager to have their day in court. They want closure.

As has been pointed out throughout this book, plenty has been written over the past several years about the impact of physician disclosure on litigation. It was mentioned earlier that health-care providers tend to shy away from telling the truth of adverse events because of fear that doing so will put them in a more vulnerable position to be sued. There is also the fear that if such information is released during a trial, it could put the physician and the health-care system for which he or she works in a very poor light.

This assumption and fear is underscored and fed by legal counsel (which may be inexperienced when it comes to medical-legal matters), as well as a hospital's risk management department. The lawyers may tell the doctors not to talk to patients; in fact, the more that doctors are able to keep quiet about an error, the better.

In truth, the silence can hurt a situation more than can disclosure or discussion. Carroll (2015), who discussed studies linking malpractice and lawsuits, concurred that a lack of communication on the physician's part is one large reason for a lawsuit. It seems as though patients and their families only want information when it comes to a mistake. Once they have that information, they're willing to forgive and let go.

A 1992 study among mothers of newborns sustaining permanent injuries who sued indicated that a third said their doctors wouldn't talk openly to them, half said their doctors tried to mislead them, and 70 percent indicated they weren't warned about long-term neurodevelopmental problems in their children (Carroll, 2015).

Another study, published two years later, examined patient

satisfaction and physicians' history in the face of malpractice suits. A doctor with a lawsuit on his or her record, regardless of the outcome, was regarded with a higher level of suspicion, even if that doctor had a sterling record otherwise. In other cases, doctors who had been through lawsuits didn't necessarily have reassuring bedside manners. Specifically, patients seeing doctors who were sued in the past were "significantly more likely to report that their doctor rushed them, did not explain reasons for tests or ignored them." It's difficult to suggest whether these doctors simply didn't care to explain reasons for tests or treatment or whether the organization for which the doctors worked wanted them to keep silent. The point here was that patients weren't given information from physicians who had been sued in the past. So silence hasn't exactly helped the position of the health-care provider when it comes to an adverse medical event. However, physicians with lawsuits on their records may come across as cold, uncaring, or uncommunicative, traits that are not necessarily desireable in the event of an adverse medical event.

Adding insult to injury, trial lawyers handling malpractice suits are forced to act on incomplete information. This is because they perceive themselves as advocates for the health-care provider and the organizaion for which he or she works, rather than mediators who are interested in getting to the bottom of a mistake and ensuring that similar mistakes don't happen again (Boothman, Imhoff, and Campbell Jr., 2012). With this outlook, the lawyer's goal is to create a case in the context of an adversarial relationship with the medical community, with the patient as the "bad guy" and the lawyer the defender of the good-hearted physician who was doing nothing more than his or her job in treating the patient. These attorneys are not being paid to be neutral or understanding. Their goal is to win on behalf of their clients.

Furthermore, these attorneys are compelled to consider the costs and benefits of taking on a particular case—as such, lawsuits are often filed even before either side understands if they have a conflict, which makes little sense (Boothman, Imhoff, and Campbell Jr., 2012). On top of this, the hospital's legal counsel, who, as mentioned earlier, may have little to no knowledge about litigation procedures, doesn't stop to analyze whether litigating each and every case is actually the best possible outcome for the health-care system. As I point out in the following, there are plenty of other options that can be used to settle disputes that don't involve trial lawyers, juries, or courtrooms. However, legal counsel, interested in keeping high billable hours, will likely not consider one of these alternative methods of dispute resolution when it comes to dealing with a frustrated patient and that patient's request for information.

Finally, the physicians themselves, told by trial lawyers to keep mum in an ongoing litigation situation, are relieved not to have to talk to angry or aggrieved patients or families. This makes sense—no one wants to be the bearer of bad news, and it is very difficult to admit on-the-job mistakes or failures, even for those who might not have physicians' larger egos. I indicated earlier that it is human nature to want to sweep these failures under the rug and hope they go away, which is part of why deny-and-defend works so effectively. The worst nightmare a physician can face is to tell a patient and his or her family, "I goofed, and here is the result."

However, that short-term relief of not having to face the injured patient and his or her angry family can come at a longer-term cost—failure of communication or, rather, the tendency not to communicate at all leads to costly legal issues. However, according to one study, plaintiffs actually end up dropping close to 59 percent of medical malpractice suits because of information accumulated during an investigation that shows the plaintiff has little or no case (Golann, 2011). Even if the plantif drops the claim, he or she is no better off than before in understanding what caused a particular medical error or mistake—and an apology is still not forthcoming.

Finally, unless a plaintiff has a lawyer who is either a medical expert or who knows medical experts, that plaintiff could be at the mercy of a defendant who is better coached. Noted Golann,

> For instance, a medical record may suggest that a required step in treatment was not taken, but a defendant may later testify persuasively in a deposition that the step was taken but simply not recorded. Or a lawyer may file suit in reliance on a expert's opinion, only to find that, as the expert sees more data, she becomes less willing to testify that malpractice occurred. (2011)

Golann discovered that other reasons a suit might be dropped include a change in the plaintiff's medical condition or a co-occurring condition that could break a causal connection. For instance, a patient who might sue over a poorly performed heart treatment could end up dying of lung cancer before the cardiac issue that led to serious injury even makes it to trial. In this situation, the lung cancer death could point to the patient's overall poor health condition, making the suit appear to be frivolous. And, once again, when such a suit is dropped, it could still be without any explanation as to what caused the poorly performed heart treatment in the first place. Certainly, it could have been because of the patient's overall poor health. But the grieving patient's family doesn't know this for a fact, which doesn't help the overall situation at all.

And finally, malpractice claims can also become weaker if the attorney in question had investigated more thoroughly before bringing suit. Sometimes, during the discovery phase of a suit, exact information might be forthcoming, which could prove that the health-care provider did everything that was required, but the end result was that the patient was injured. To reiterate, medicine is a dangerous profession, with outcomes not necessarily assured of always being positive. Whenever a surgeon cuts into a patient, there is the risk of injury or death. As such, there is no guarantee that a patient will come out of a surgery better than when he or she went under the knife. If a patient's family understands that everything was done to save a patient (and the exact reason why a patient might have died), the family likely won't want to participate in costly litigation.

What is at issue with litigation is the lack of information pertaining to an adverse medical event. This, in turn, has led Boothman et al. (2012) to conclude that "the dearth of communication among caregivers, patients and trial lawyers affords little chance that the parties will achieve an understanding sort of litigation." No matter how litigation might end—either in a dropped case or one that makes it all the way to trial and a jury decision—understanding between the two parties involved with the litigation is likely to be nonexistent. In fact, an adversarial relationship will likely be in place over the long term.

Golann also weighed in on the problems with litigating a medical error, suggesting that the way to avoid dropped claims (and to do a better job of resolving cases) is to change the malpractice culture, to make it less about "us against them." He pointed out that each side in a malpractice case is typically adversarial; the sides fear that the other will take advantage of openness or reasonableness, meaning there is a lack of both. Any honest admission of error is considered a weapon that can be used in the opposition's toolkit, especially if a case makes it all the way to trial. As a result of this assumption, medical insurers, health-care providers, institutions, and defense lawyers fall back into deny-and-defend, only disclosing bits and pieces of information that the court rules require and making low initial settlement offers (Golann, 2011; see also Boothman et al., 2009). It's little wonder that plaintiffs bringing suits against doctors and hospitals for injuries during treatment become that much more frustrated.

Finally, when it comes to litigation, trial lawyers aren't necessarily in the business of taking a deep dive into why errors took place or what to do to prevent those errors from occurring again. Rather, their responsibility is to defend their client, no matter what the mistake was, even if the error could have been preventable. What the trial lawyer is doing, in a sense, is defending clinical care that shouldn't be defended in the first place. The litigation system is also set up to ensure that health-care institutions don't examine causes or even their own practices that might have led to an adverse medical event. Rather, the trial system is set up to protect those institutions from adversarial relationships from the plaintiff. As Beth Daley Ullem understood in her own experience, the hospital at which her newborn son died had had similar events in the past. Rather than examine those events and take steps to ensure they didn't happen again, the hospital circled the wagons, turned a silence to her questions, and continued with its wrongful practices.

Yet the secretive approach of deny-and-defend and the adversarial stance a hospital or health-care organization can take in light of a medical error can also backfire. When Daley Ullem's son died, her only goal was to find out what prompted the medical error that caused the death. The last thing on her mind was a lawsuit—she didn't want to go through the time, expense, or emotions that such an action would require. She was, in fact, up front about her inclination not to sue the doctors or hospital; all she wanted to know was how "you're going to improve and protect families" (Smith, 2019). However, Ullem Daley was stonewalled from the start, meaning no investigation, no answers, and no assurance of improvement. Adding insult to the injury of her loss, she went on to say that the event in question was even hidden from the hospital's quality department. "To me, that was going from error to insult," she commented.

Daley Ullem also pointed out that she wasn't after information to use as part of a lawsuit to hammer the physicians or hospitals, noting that, "I think people are remarkably forgiving if you say right away, 'here's what happened, here's what we're going to improve, and we're not going to hide from you.'"

However, what the story doesn't suggest is whether, following the lawsuit and Daley Ullem's victory, the hospital changed its ways, put into place an error-reporting system, or began a system of disclosure, with apologies built in. The story didn't say if that hospital, realizing the error of its ways, initiated change in its policies, allowing its physicians to acknowledge errors when they happen and helping patients by presenting information as to why an adverse event took place. Nor did the story suggest that this hospital's culture of deny-and-defend was eradicated following the lawsuit. The chances are pretty good that, following the litigation, nothing changed for this institution. It's likely that the hospital continued its practices of closing ranks around errors, not examining mistakes to determine how improvements could take place and keeping patient safety in mind. As such, the chances are good that the next time a mother loses a newborn baby to poor institutional practices and that mother is stonewalled in finding information as to why, the hospital and its team will close ranks. This, in turn, will likely lead to another costly lawsuit, another multimillion-dollar verdict, and another mother saying, "I didn't want to sue; I simply wanted information about what happened."

Clearly, the litigation system, as it currently stands, doesn't really provide any method for a physician or health-care system to honestly take a look at its mistakes and learn from them and, in conclusion, to help ensure that similar mistakes don't take place. It doesn't provide a vehicle either for full disclosure or for ensuring proper apologies. In fact, litigation is the absolute worst tool that can be used for dealing with medical mistakes or encouraging disclosure of such mistakes, for the following reasons.

1) Litigation tends to breed an adversarial relationship between the plaintiff, who only wants answers, and the defendant,

who is part of a deny-and-defend culture that refuses to admit any wrongdoing or mistakes.

2) Litigation is spearheaded by attorneys who, for the most part, don't truly understand medical malpractice or why errors take place. These attorneys are only focused on one thing: making sure their clients are protected at all costs.

3) Such an atmosphere means information is automatically disclosed or is only disclosed based on court rulings. Even if a case makes it to trial, there is no guarantee that a plaintiff is going to receive a satisfactory explanation as to why a particular event took place, thereby increasing the frustration level when it comes to understanding the cause of a medical error.

4) The litigation process is geared to protect poor practices and recurring mistakes rather than to improve them. Whether a defendant wins or loses, there is no effort to uncover why an error took place or what needs to be done to prevent it in the future. The process of litigation doesn't allow an organization to take a careful look at what prompted a medical error in the first place and to make necessary improvements.

5) Litigation prevents a health-care provider from apologizing or showing empathy, for fear that such behavior could end up harming that individual (or the hospital for which he or she works) through evidence. Even if a physician is trained in the art of an appropriate apology, he or she will be cautioned not to say a word to the patient. As a result, the process of forgiveness is stymied with neither patient nor physician being able to move forward.

In short, using litigation as a means of extracting information in the face of a medical mistake is not the most efficient way. Many times, however, it can be the only way for an injured party to obtain satisfaction, especially when dealing with an organization that is involved with deny-and-defend practices.

The good news here is that, in an effort to spur tort reform and to reduce malpractice claims, alternative dispute resolution (ADR) techniques are available. When used correctly, these tools can help parties come together, discuss the issues, and hopefully come to a satisfactory resolution of an issue.

# ADR, MEDIATION, AND ARBITRATION

IN BETWEEN THE STONE WALL OF SILENCE FOLLOWING A medical error and a hoped-for and potential full disclosure through a lawsuit and the courts is a concept known as alternative dispute resolution, or ADR. While the goal of this thesis is to determine whether a doctor's apology can help defer legal action in the face of an adverse medical event, a discussion of ADR techniques is necessary to demonstrate the idea of full disclosure in response to a medical error. This is because such techniques provide solutions to outright lawsuits when it comes to settling issues a patient or his or her family might have when it comes to medical treatment, without incurring the expense and time necessary for a trial by jury. Such techniques allow the patient or patient's family to meet with the physicians and the organization's staff directly, discuss the situation in a rational manner, obtain information pertinent to the case, and then determine the best outcome and compensation, depending on the circumstances.

ADR can help both parties avoid the courts and trial by jury by focusing on creating solutions to resolving harm and disputes; however, creative solutions could be limited or restricted by the courts.

## ◆ Defining Alternative Dispute Resolution

In taking a deeper dive into the concept of ADR, we find that this is a catchall phrase for techniques, outside of a court of law, that can be used to help put the brakes on medical malpractice lawsuits. Because they can be used outside the litigation system, ADR allows health-care providers and the health-care systems in which they operate to acknowledge openly when errors have occurred, while offering reasonable compensation to the injured patients and their families if called for (Kass and Rose, 2016). Basically, ADR allows patients and physicians to move from a defensive posture—a "battle" strategy that is common within a litigation situation—and into a faciliated, directed conversation with the ultimate goal of conflict resolution being that physicians who are confronted with medical errors tend to be defensive and feel as though their practice or reputation is taking a hit. However, patients who are stonewalled by no acknowledgment of error tend to feel abandoned and betrayed. Use of ADR techniques can help break through this impasse and help the physician and patient come to a better understanding and agreement as to what actually took place.

As mentioned earlier, the collection of ADR techniques can include mediation and arbitration (discussed earlier), as well as early apology and pretrial screenings (Sohn and Bal, 2012). I'll discuss mediation and arbitration in more detail in the following sections, but I wanted to touch on early apologies and pretrial screenings as ADR techniques.

Though physicians have been cautioned not to say a word in the case of pending litigation, apologies during an ADR process can have the potential to facilitate discussion and resolution, as long as the injured party thinks he or she has been treated fairly and whether he or she attributes fault to the particular health-care provider or offender (McMichael, 2018). Basically, the issue here is fair versus unfair treatment—apologies can really only work in a situation in which a victim feels as though he or she is being treated fairly throughout the ADR process. Furthermore, from a search of research pertaining to early apologies versus legal cases, it was found that such programs reported a 50 percent to 67 percent success rate in avoiding litigation, as well as substantial reductions when it came to the amount paid per claim (Sohn and Bal, 2012). The early disclosure and apology isn't as formal as mediation and boils down to a meeting between the two parties involved in an adverse medical event, during which they discuss the conflict and achieve some type of resolution. These exchanges can be prompted by programs specifically designed to facilitate apologies, which I will discuss in greater detail in an upcoming section.

Another ADR technique is known as pretrial screenings, which represent informal screenings prior to formal litigation. More than half the states in the United States require pretrial screenings before a case goes to active trial. Such screenings are conducted by a neutral party who assesses the relative strengths and merits of each party's case and determines whether the information present can provide enough reason for going to trial. This can be effective in a medical malpractice case, because there tends to be a high number of cases in the field that don't really merit trial. Many malpractice suits, in fact, don't even make it to trial and are dropped by the plaintiff. This makes sense—if the reason why claimants decide to file suit against a physician or organization is simply to obtain information about a mistake (to break through the wall of silence), there might not be enough "meat" in the case for a full-blown trial by jury.

Furthermore, a reason for the high number of meritless claims is because plaintiffs can often become confused about what does and doesn't constitute medical negligence. One issue that I introduced up front is that the practice of medicine, by its very nature, carries a number of inherent risks, such as infection, bleeding, pain, and even death. Plaintiffs might not understand that certain complications can be a part of treatment and either experiencing pain or injury resulting from medical care (or having a family member who is expericing pain and injury from said care) might be unexpected, or possibly, those potential complications weren't explained up front before treatment started. A patient, or family, who wants redress from a medical error (especially in the face of silence when attempting to obtain more information about that mistake) might decide to file a lawsuit, simply because they feel that's the way to go in an attempt to ease pain and suffering. Unfortunately, personal injury attorneys are all too happy to back such a suit; if they win, or even if the case is settled out of court, there can be a nice payoff. A pretrial screening can help steer plaintiffs toward more fruitful means of redress and information gathering, such as mediation or even arbitration.

### ◆ Mediation

Mediation increasingly is becoming a tool used to help facilitate communication between patients and physicians following an adverse medical event or error (Liebman, 2011). Mediation is defined as a "confidential, voluntary process in which an impartial third party—the mediator—helps the participants negotiate their differences and either craft a mutually acceptable solution or decide to deal with their problems in some other manner" (Liebman and Hyman, 2004). Mediation is based on three core values: autonomy, informed decision-making, and confidentiality. These three core values are essential when it comes to providing comfort, both to the patient who feels he or she might have been wronged and to the physician, who might think he is being judged.

The idea behind mediation is the belief that most people involved with a conflict have the ability, given the right setting and access to the right information, to select resolutions that meet their needs. It assumes that, given the right situation, adversarial individuals can be reasonable, if they hear the other person's side of things. Basically, adding a mediator can add value to a dispute, as he or she can be a guide or coach to help the disputants move from position-based negotiations to interest-based negotiations. In other words, a skilled and trained mediator can go beyond the emotional scenarios on both sides of the table, add calm to the procedings, and ensure that both parties come to conclusions that are in their own best interests. With a disinterested third party (the mediator) involved in the proceedings, resolution becomes that much easier, because the mediator has no bias and no "skin in the game."

Furthermore, in a mediation setting, participants can request and offer information; the mediator, in fact, encourages the exchange of information. This is a very important concept; I've already outlined that the wish of patients and families when it comes to an adverse medical event is to determine why the event occurred in the first place. The free flow of information during the mediation process can help the victims affected by a medical mistake better understand what took place and that it won't happen again, meaning the victims won't need to resort to a discovery process through a lawsuit.

As for the mediators, they spend a great deal of time in initial training and ongoing education to develop the attributes necessary to ensure that both parties walk away from the process satisfied. They are required to develop active listening and conflict resolution skills that are necessary when it comes to conducting any kind of disclosure and informational conversations. It's important to understand that these skills aren't acquired overnight but rather require a great deal of practice and continuous use to be maintained. This is why, more often than not, mediation needs to be handled by a trained mediator rather than a health-care professional or hospital / health-care system executive. Health-care providers' time is already at a premium when it comes to their daily activities. They don't have the time necessary to develop mediation skills, especially as they aren't likely going to need them all that often. Because of this, it makes sense to bring an outside person into a mediation process and to have that individual supervise the procedings.

Furthermore, mediators, by nature of their purpose, are neutral; they aren't emotionally invested in the outcome of a particular medical situation, unlike a patient or patient's family or doctor. Additionally, mediators aren't part of the organization that is involved with the adverse event and don't know either of the parties involved in the scenario.

There are various mediation models when it comes to resolving medical practice disputes. One such model, introduced by Carole Liebman and Chris Stern Hyman, proposes the following steps:

- training the communicators
- planning the discussions
- providing emotional support to the health-care providers
- resolving the claims
- mediating dispute resolution

The authors felt that this particular model would help health-care providers better communicate more effectively with patients following an adverse medical event, as well as learn from their mistakes and arrive at a cost-effective resolution of valid claims. The model was also used in the Pew Demonstration Mediation and ADR Project, which focused on an exchange of information and methods taken to avoid similar errors in the future.

The Demonstration Mediation and ADR Project came about in 2002 with the goal of studying the value of mediation and open communication concerning adverse events as a potential tool to avoid costly, long-term, and bitter litigation. The demonstration project involved three hospitals in eastern Pennsylvania; while the authors, at the time, were reluctant to note that the program could be extrapolated to other areas and actually reduce litigation and costs, they did allow that if disclosure is made with compassion and includes an appropriate apology and a fair offer of compensation (along with steps to avoid similar harm), "we predict that litigation will decrease and patient safety will improve."

However, Liebman and Hyman also pointed out that, even with an ideal mediation model, an entrenched culture of deny-and-defend can be dificult to break through, pointing out that strong leadership will be required to change institutional and professional responses to an adverse medical event.

Outside of the Pew Demonstration Mediation and ADR Project, can mediation, overall, help avoid a long, drawn-out litigation process? Two studies focused on this very question, one of which examined cases brought against the New York City Health and Hospitals Corp (HHC), and another that detailed Mediating Suits against Hospitals (MeSH) (Hyman, Liebman, Schechter, and Sage, 2010).

Overall, the majority of the plaintiffs who attended the mediations in both studies found it to be a positive experience. The attorneys, perhaps unsurprisingly, weren't as enamoured with it—those responding to the MeSH study indicated they would have preferred an evaluative approach to mediation.

Both studies, however, did find that the mediation processes were time-efficient; with the HHC study, attorneys estimated they spent approximately one-tenth as much time preparing for mediation as for litigation. In the MeSH study, lawyers reported three to ten hours of preparation for mediation versus the estimates of one hundred hours or more when it came to ligitation and trial preparation. Discovery, in the meantime, was completed in ten of twenty MeSH cases and partially completed in eight others—however, there was no correlation between the stage in litigation and likelihood of settlement.

However, the MeSH study noted that while mediation did provide savings by shortening the litigation process and that the plantiffs and attorneys were satisfied with the results, major challenges continue to stand in the way of experiencing the full benefits of mediation. One problem cited by the study was lack of physician participation in the mediation process (Hyman, Liebman, Schechter, and Sage, 2010). The lack of physician presence means this type of mediation deprives both sides of "the opportunity for healing, understanding, forgiveness and repair of broken relationships and failed communication." Another issue here and one that has been mentioned throughout this book is that mediation, apologies, or any other resolution models are only as good as the organizations that administer them. If an organization is not interested in using mediation as a tool for dispute resolution, it won't be very effective. Specifically, change is necessary, so that medical leaders, hospital administrators, and malpractice insurers get rid of their suspicions of the tort system sufficiently to consider medical errors and adverse events as learning opportunities rather than a vehicle by which to point blame. Furthermore, these organizations need to hire and retain lawyers who consider mediation to be an opportunity to solve problems and improve care, while showing compassion, as opposed to viewing mediation as a lesser tool to resolution than outright litigation. Otherwise, according to Hyman et al., "the singular focus on monetary remedies characteristic of lawyer-to-lawyer negotiation will continue to contaminate mediation," with the inability to focus on nonmonetary remedies.

Still, both studies demonstrated that mediation can help reduce costs, provide plaintiffs with the opportunity to be heard and to share their side of an issue, and, just as important, allow defendants to obtain the necessary information to help improve quality of care—at least, as long as physicians are allowed to participate in the process. Noted Liebman,

> If parties make use of mediation to reach settlement closer in time to the adverse event, defendants will

realize significant savings in litigation costs, plaintiffs will receive compensation sooner when they need it most, and plaintiffs' lawyers will still receive adequate compensation for their work.

Furthermore, the mediation type used in the Pew model was desgned to encourage claims settlements as soon as both parties had adequate information to evaluate the case and to give the participants enough opportunity to consider noneconomic concerns. Through this model, the mediator encourages an exchange of information, while facilitating discussions about how such errors can be avoided in the future. Liebman and Hyman suggest that parties should mediate cases sooner rather than later, after a claim has been filed and before "expensive and hostility escalating discovery has been conducted."

And there is indication that the use of mediation means savings to the tune of $50,000 per claim, with a 90 percent satisfaction rate among both claimants and defendants (Sohn and Bal, 2012).

There are, however, times during which mediation might not be a helpful tool. For example, when the future costs of long-term care are not yet clear, mediation might not work. This is a definite issue; depending on the nature of an error or injury, the patient might require more medical care, the extent to which is not known at the time of a proposed mediation session.

Mediation is also not appropriate if a plaintiff isn't emotionally ready to consider a settlement or there are concerns that information is being withheld or is not yet available. As mentioned before, victims of adverse medical events do want information to help with closure.

There are those, however, who feel as though they might want revenge through a full-fledged trial by jury. In this particular case, mediation won't be effective, as the claimant in question wouldn't be ready to accept any explanation from the doctor in question.

The conclusion here is that, while mediation can be a helpful tool when it comes to airing issues between patients and physicians, it isn't necessarily the right tool for all specific cases. Whether mediation is successful depends on the willingness of both parties to participate in a calm, reasoned discussion and whether information can be freely released to the patient or his or her family. Still, mediation does offer a viable tool for a calm resolution, presided over by a third-party mediator who is trained in resolving dispute outcomes.

### ◆ Arbitration

Both mediation and arbitration employ a neutral third party to oversee the process, and both can be legally binding (FindLaw, 2019). However, while mediation typically relies on a single, trained mediator (not a legal expert) who is responsible for spearheading discussions between plaintiff and defendant, arbitration is typically conducted with a panel of several arbitrators, who take on the role of judges, make decisions based on evidence, and then provide written opinions, which can be either binding or nonbinding. The panelists, more often than not, are legal experts, either retired judges or attorneys.

Claimants and accused are each allowed to select an arbitrator, with the two arbitrators then selecting a third. The mediator, in contrast, does not judge cases but, rather, helps facilitate discussion and (hopefully) eventual resolution of the dispute. The benefits of arbitrating medical malpractice disputes have included the quality of the decision-makers, speed of resolution, and reduced litigation expenses (Larson, 2016). The point here is that, by involving neutral specialists (rather than lay juries) to decide medical tort cases, the results are likely to be more accurate. Another benefit to arbitration versus trial by jury is that the former means a jury doesn't have to be educated about medical practice and science.

For instance, an analysis of 1,452 litigated malpractice claims throughout the United States pointed out the average time from the opening of a medical malpractice claim to its closing was three years (Larson, 2016). But in examining 604 disputes between managed care organization Kaiser Permanente and its members, arbitrated disputes closed, on average, in less than one year.

However, there are serious questions as to whether arbitration is of benefit in an adverse medical event scenario or even when it comes to avoiding malpractice suits. On the one hand, no one argues that arbitration can be a useful tool when it comes to diverting a medical error case from a lengthy and expensive trial (Staszak, 2019). On the other hand, arbitration isn't conducted by a sympathetic, trained mediator but, rather, by a panel of what could be perceived as cold-hearted legal experts who might not be sympathetic to the plight of a patient who suffered from a medical mistake. There are also concerns of bias, namely that the defendants in an arbitration scenario are "repeat players," in other words, medical practitioners who have been involved with arbitration before, meaning that the decisions coming down from these panels might be based more on favoritism than concepts of fairness or what is right. Noted Staszak, many of the cost-saving features that make arbitration an attractive alternative to litigation are premised on the asssumption that a nonjudicial actor will rule fairly on a claim, using a record, that is often solely compiled by the defendant physician.

She also criticizes the repeat players, pointing out that these defendants, skilled in the arbitration system, are able to select arbitrators "who will be favorable to their position." In using Kaiser Permanente as an example, she points out that managed care organizations, in particular, are able to manipulate arbitration to their point of view. Staszak's focus is on private arbitration, but it is a concern that needs to be considered if using this as a tool to resolve medical disputes, rather than considering a costly legal trial.

But Larson points out, first and foremost, that physicians generally don't serve as arbitrators and that Kaiser Permanente's arbitration process requires that the arbitrators be members of the State Bar of California or retired state or federal judges. Unlike Staszak's belief of favoritism, a panel full of lawyers could mean trouble for the physicians—it's a well-known fact that doctors tend to not like, or trust, attorneys. As such, Larson notes that few should be surprised "when physicians hesitate to place their professional futures in the hands of a single, or even a panel, of three attorney arbitrators." In such a case, interestingly enough, physicians might actually prefer trial by jury to arbitration. At least they have a fighting chance of acquittal with a jury.

Furthermore, while arbitration can be less costly than taking a case to trial, the claimant will still have costs, in the form of up-front fees and out-of-pocket expenses necessary to pay for the arbitration panelists, discovery, and even expert witnesses. Costs are less likely to be an issue for physicians, as they will probably be covered by malpractice insurance.

Also unlike Staszak, Larson believes that arbitration better serves patient claimants than physicians. While patients do face up-front costs when it comes to arbitration, physicians feel as though they risk more, namely, their reputations and self-image, through an arbitration process. For example, if a physician wants to vindicate his or her reputation, a compromise forum, such as arbitration, doesn't allow this to happen. Furthermore, rather than potentially clearing a physician's name, as can happen in a trial-by-jury situation, the very nature of arbitration compromise means the physician is believed to have done something wrong, until proven otherwise. Litigation, Larson said, can help clear a physician's reputation, if the physician wins the day. Arbitration does not.

The reason why arbitration is discussed in this book is because many medical practices and health-care organizations have arbitration built into their contracts with patients, as an alternative to filing suit against a physician. In addition, arbitration can be a helpful tool when there is a specific and evidentary point of disagreement, especially when it comes to a complex issue of science (Sohn and Bal, 2012).

Still, use of arbitration to determine the outcome of of an adverse medical event is not necessarily embraced by either scholars or the medical community, given the potential for bias, on the one hand, and the tense relationship between doctors and attorneys, on the other. Throw in the up-front costs to claimants, and arbitration isn't necessarily an ideal solution for either side, especially when it comes to understanding the reasons behind a medical error. Arbitration only decides court issues without a court trial. It doesn't necessarily provide an avenue to full disclosure or even organizational claim in the face of a medical error.

### ◆ ADR in Light of Medical Error

In the preceding section, I went into detail about various methods of alternative dispute resolution and their use to reduce the potential for litigation and malpractice suits. While ADR techniques don't necessarily fit into the "apology" mode, if handled correctly, they can be helpful in opening the channels of communication between claimants and respondents, even through arbitration. Many times, the airing of grievances—on both sides—can provide both parties with an understanding about what each side is feeling and believing. This could, in turn, create a path to an amicable settlement that benefits both sides. And ADR methods, when handled correctly, can help take out the confrontational stance that prevents meaningful discussion or settlement when it comes to physician or health-care organization error.

Getting back to the original thesis, however, ADR tools rarely, if ever, focus on apologizing as part of a disclosure process and whether apologizing can help reduce the chances of litigation in the face of a medical error or adverse event. In the next section, I'll discuss communication-and-resolution programs, which are geared to provide immediate disclosure, apologies, and settlements, and determine the effectiveness of such a technique.

# COMMUNICATION-AND-RESOLUTION PROGRAMS

SINCE *TO ERR IS HUMAN* WAS PUBLISHED, MEDICAL ERROR disclosure has become a very hot topic, leading a variety of healthcare systems to draft policies and committees to address issues such as disclosures to patients, their families, and other interested parties (Taft, 2005). And, as I've mentioned throughout this book, within that particular issue of disclosure is the use of the apology for communicating unexpected and unanticipated outcomes to medical events.

It's interesting to note specifics about what happens when physicians apologize for errors—in the proper way. David Hilfiker, an American writer and physician, penned an essay in 1986 in which he discussed mistakes he had made while working as a doctor in Minnesota. At that time, he pointed out that acknowledgment of the error to patients and their families provided a better connection between humans, as well as helped to pave the way toward forgiveness (Hilfiker, 1984). He also added, however, that physicians are exempted from the process because mistakes in the medical arena can cause severe harm to patients. It's been mentioned before that physicians hold a great deal of power over their patients, in many cases, the power of life and death. As such, mistakes can create havoc within patients' lives and those of their families. Additionally, physicians have felt the fear of the consequences from an apology, in a scenario which Hilfiker dubbed an "intolerable dilemma."

Hilfiker's discussion addressed Wu's "second victim" scenario, one in which physicians who are not allowed to, or might not know how to, apologize suffer from guilt and shame resulting from the medical error. It also supports Allan and McKillop's contention that patients and families who have been wronged really want to forgive but might be prevented from doing so because of a deny-and-defend culture that prohibits any explanation or apology resulting from an adverse medical ereror. Disclosure and admission of remorse can alleviate the physician's second victim situation, while, as Hilfiker noted, helping to pave the path toward forgiveness and helping the physician to heal from his or her error, as well.

Overall, apologies can help decrease feelings of frustration and anger on behalf of the patients and their families; if left unchecked, that frustration and anger can drive those harmed by a medical error to file lawsuits (Ackerman, 2018). Disclosure benefits could include increased transparency, support for clinicians responsible for or facing adverse events, and enhanced patient safety because of the examination of errors.

A more formalized approach to a physician apology involves communication-and-resolution programs.

### ◆ Rick Boothman, Defense Attorney

During the late 1990s, defense attorney Rick Boothman found himself defending a surgeon whose patient experienced a postoperative infection (Smith, 2019). Said patient sued the doctor, and the case went to trial. Between evidence collection, depositions, and docket scheduling, six years passed between the initial suit and the trial; during that time, the two parties said nothing to each other. Boothman thought that more than half decade of silence bizarre, pointing out that "One day you take someone's life into your hands, and the next day you're not talking to them?"

The verdict was rendered in the surgeon's favor, and the jury departed. The woman who had sued turned to her doctor, saying, "If I had known everything I heard in this courtroom, I never would have sued you." In other words, the information the plaintiff heard during the trial told her what she needed to know and softened her stance as to the surgeon's side of the issue. It's not likely the attorney representing the plaintiff would have been as sympathetic, so the trial did go to a verdict, meaning a lot of expense and time was spent on something that should have been resolved with a simple, and honest, conversation.

Boothman, observing this, came to an epiphany, namely that if people actually talked more, honestly and openly, following a medical error, it was likely that lawsuits and litigations could be decreased. This led to the concept of communication-and-resolution programs. Under such a program, a physician, hospital, or healthcare system discloses a medical error at once, the causes of it, and what will change because of it. The CRP also provides reasonable compensation, agreeable by both sides. It could be said that the CRP is an early-on apology for making a mistake.

Before going into this in more detail, let's examine the purpose of compensation offers. In some situations, it's not uncommon for patients to decline early compensation offers in response to injury from a medical procedure. This doesn't have much to do with the money or how much patients and their families think they can get from the courts, but more because money isn't necessarily the major issue when it comes to filing litigation against perceived wrongdoing. The major issue, as has been stressed throughout this book, is information—why the medical error occurred and what will happen to ensure that a similar error won't take place in the future. Early compensation offers can sometimes omit all this information, which is why claimants could reject those offers until they have more information.

Because of the nature of their disclosure, CRPs don't seem to have this problem—everything is up front, early in the process (in most cases, almost immediately after a medical mistake has taken place), so the wronged party understands what has occurred and what will be corrected. Under this scenario, when compensation is offered, it's more likely to be accepted, as the claimant has that information.

However, it somewhat goes without saying, in the face of "deny-and-defend," that Boothman's idea for transparency wasn't accepted with open arms by the medical community. Even to this day, the culture among many health-care organizations is that clinicians continue to be worried if they issue a statement of fault, they'll be blamed for something, while health-care leaders continue to believe attorneys, who forecast that CRP will mean more malpractice suits and potential financial ruin. Then there is the fear from the legal community that attorneys, who bill by the hour, will be harmed by CRP. After all, no litigation means no billings. There have been no studies, however, to prove that any of these concerns are realized. Later on in this book, I'll provide case studies about CRP and apology programs that have successfully reduced malpractice lawsuits. In all my research, however, I've not found evidence that health-care systems implementing CRP programs have actually seen an increase in medical lawsuits or malpractice litigation.

In fact, research and studies show that communication-and-resolution programs can have a positive impact on medical liability processes and outcomes (Lambert, et al., 2016). In one study at the University of Illinois Chicago Medical Center (which I will focus on in more detail in the following chapter), it was found that the implementation of a "Seven Pillars" strategy involving disclosure and communication doubled the number of incident reports, while halving the number of legal claims and reducing legal fees. Additionally, the approach reduced legal fees and total costs per claim, settlement amounts, and self-insurance amounts.

Another study noted that when the health-care staff was willing to apologize for and resolve medical errors through a collaborativ e-communication-and-resolution program (CCRP), they realized a significant decrease in defense costs, legal claims, and liability costs (Ackerman, 2018; see also LeCraw, et al., 2018).

How about when it comes to disclosing others' errors? It can be difficult for a practitioner to willingly admit errors perpetrated by a colleague. If a clinician wasn't directly involved in an adverse event, he or she might not have enough firsthand knowledge of the event (Gallagher, et al., 2013). Then there are the peer groups—loyalty and solidarity can sometimes mean silence when an adverse event takes place. However, a culture in which transparency and disclosure are a regular part of health-care practice can help break that wall of silence and, rather than casting blame or throwing a colleague under the bus, can help in understanding the causes of a particular problem and ensuring that those problems don't happen again. In such a situation, it is, of course, encumbent on the physician to obtain information on what happened, before disclosing that information to a patient or patient's family.

Before continuing, it's important to realize that apology programs and CRPs are not the same as ADR techniques, especially mediation and arbitration. Certainly, all these tools are useful for potentially avoiding malpractice litigation in the face of an adverse medical event. But they are different in nature. CRP, by its very nature, involves prompt disclosure, explanation, an apology, and compensation. It could be said that mediation and arbitration might be the next step, in the event that the patient or patient's family isn't satisfied with the results of the CRP efforts. Despite the good intentions of a CRP program, it might not be the right fit for all situations.

It's been found, however, that mediators can be helpful to the CRP process. For instance, in states that don't have "apology laws" or statutes that protect CRP communications, a mediator can be helpful by bringing skills—such as active listening—to help diffuse any potentially volatile situations (Supra, 2019). This is because mediators have the skills that other participants could lack, as dispute resolution isn't their full-time job.

Mediation, as mentioned earlier, is helpful when it comes to research and discovery. Furthermore, research and discovery are helpful when it comes to any kind of apology or resolution program. These can be valuable assets for a CRP plan.

In all, the purpose of disclosure programs is to provide open communication between the health-care provider and patient or patient's family in the case of an adverse medical event. Because the physician's focus is, first and foremost, a professional and personal duty to the patient (not to mention an obligation to disclose, according to the ethicists), disclosure programs can help ensure that trust is built between the perpetrator of the medical error and the individual harmed by it. This, in turn, can, in most cases, decrease the potential of litigation. As pointed out earlier, litigation does little to help a situation, except add time, cost, and emotional stress to both sides of the issue.

### ◆ Anatomy of a CRP—CANDOR

While there are a variety of CRPs in existence, it's best to examine one released by the Agency for Healthcare Research and Quality, which is called the "Communication and Optimal Resolution Toolkit," or CANDOR, for short (Boothman, 2016; see also AHRQ, 2016). This toolkit was tested in fourteen hospitals and across three US health systems, and it was found to be successful in prompting disclosure of adverse medical events, while avoiding potential litigation costs. The toolkit ranges from obtaining organizational buy-in and support for a hospital or health-care organization's disclosure model to preparing for program implementation, to response and disclosure, to organizational learning and sustainability.

The toolkit itself is broken into eight modules that are used to teach health-care organizations about the CANDOR process. Furthermore, the toolkit defines a CANDOR event as one that "involves unexpected patient harm ... physical, emotional, or financial." The toolkit points out that the CANDOR process is triggered, even when a cause for the event isn't known.

The following represents what typically happens in the event of an adverse medical event and how the CANDOR program works when an adverse medical event takes place.

| Deny-and-Defend Response | CANDOR Response |
| --- | --- |
| Little to no involvement of, or communication with, patients and families | Patient and family involvement are extensive and ongoing; communication is transparent and open |
| Reporting by clinicians is delayed or absent | Clinicians are encouraged to immediately report the error/event |
| Assesses blame to physician and/or nurse for the medical error | Event analysis incorporates Just Culture, systems, and human error when determining the cause for the error |
| Care for the clinicians is frequently absent | Supports immediate and ongoing support for clinicians following an event |

| Patient/family rarely receives monetary compensation and only if they file, and prevail, on a malpractice claim | Health-care organization proactively addresses the patient and family needs and offers reasonable compensation, when warranted |
| --- | --- |
| Little is learned; clinicians and systems aren't retrained following an adverse medical event | Promotes value of disseminating lessons learned and solutions to prevent similar harm in the future |

CANDOR and similar disclosure programs are geared toward 1) immediate reporting of an adverse event; 2) ongoing communication and support of the patient and family following the event; 3) ongoing support of the clinician or practitioner throughout the process; 4) event investigation and analysis conducted by a core team, which is responsible for interviewing and collecting information (as well as telling the billing department to hold the patient's bill until the investigation is completed); 5) determining causal factors for the event and whether standard of care was met; and 6) developing a plan of action to be shared with the patient, family, providers, and insurance carriers. Once this process is completed, the final component of the CANDOR program involves resolution, which can only take place after the investigation and analysis are concluded (AHRQ, 2016). The resolution phase not only determines compensation for the patient and family but also engages them in discussions and commentary about preventing recurrence of similar harm events.

# CAN DISCLOSURE WORK? CASE STUDIES

THE BEST WAY TO DETERMINE IF DISCLOSURE OF ADverse events is effective is by putting the theory to test in the real world. Certainly, it seems as though early disclosure checks boxes of honesty, transparency, and something patients want. And studies reveal that early disclosure can have a drastic effect on the number of lawsuits issued in the face of an adverse medical event. In this section, the focus will be on specific CRP disclosure programs and whether they have actually led to a decrease in malpractice claims and lawsuits.

◆ **University of Michigan**

When discussing the disclosure of adverse events, both when it comes to models and training in doing so and the impact on malpractice suits, the literature, more often than not, turns to the University of Michigan Health System (UMHS) as the pioneer in breaking through the deny-and-defend focus and more into a culture of honesty and transparency. This is because UMHS was one of the first health-care systems to implement a CRP program and has definitely made it work.

Much like other health-care systems in the late twentieth century, UMHS had an adversarial relationship with the legal system, as well as with patients who tried to question errors resulting from adverse medical events or tried to seek information on what caused those errors in the first place (Boothman, Imhoff, and Campbell Jr., 2012). The system became self-insured in 1985, internally controlling its defenses—litigation management was under the umbrella of the health system's legal office, which contained lawyers from the university's Office of General Counsel. In other words, these attorneys had little to no experience when it came to medical malpractice. At the same time, UMHS had struck relationships with trial law firms, with the idea that competition would mean more favorable hourly rates. The lawyers of these firms, responsible for investigating cases, retaining independent experts, and preparing defense, were overseen by lawyers or risk managers with no personal trial experience when it came to malpractice lawsuits. And, before 2001, trial lawyers (with little to no experience in medical malpractice) "defended the vast majority of the UMHS' claims, consistent with the expected deny-and-defend approach."

According to Boothman and his colleagues, the UMHS setup was perfectly suited for deny-and-defend, with two committees reviewing claims at the end of the malpractice process, typically right before the cases were scheduled to start trial. One committee focused on medical defense strategies, while the other, a traditional claims committee, approved the settlements or the trial decisions. Not much was disclosed in the early part of the process, however, and that was by choice. The end result of this system was that most decisions occurred near the end of lengthy (and costly) litigation, while most cases were settled, not tried, despite the merits of the claims. This not only prevented apologies when it came to perceived wrongdoing but also didn't provide patients or their families with explanations when something went wrong in the course of treatment.

Perhaps unsurprisingly, by the end of the twentieth century, UMHS found the deny-and-defend system it had in place to be unsustainable. Leaders running the organization realized that relying on trial lawyers as a response to patients' injuries put UMHS in chronic fights when it came to the majority of claims. That fight response meant a consistent adversarial relationship with patients, versus attempting to help them, while determining what went wrong and what caused an error or adverse event in the first place.

After doing a great deal of internal soul-searching, research, and study, UMHS realized the following:

- UMHS didn't require litigation to determine the difference between reasonable and unreasonable care.
- Litgation needed to be avoided, given the high financial, emotional, and productivity costs. Litigation, in fact, should be considered as the last resort in an injury or adverse medical event situation.
- Settling clinical cases in which care was reasonable (or didn't cause injury) left clinical staff demoralized.
- Defending care below the UMHS standard of practice ended up creating significant unnecessary costs, while undermining institutional quality and safety culture goals.

During 2001, in response to this internal research, three principles were circulated for approval among those in the UMHS claims management:

- Compensate patients quickly and fairly when unreasonable medical care caused injury.
- If care was reasonable or didn't adversely affect the clinical outcome, support the health-care providers and organization.
- Reduce patient injuries—and claims—by learning through patients' experiences.

In working with the UMHS approach, Boothman et al. further pointed out that the three principles led to a transparency and honesty approach, which can be boiled down to a handful of specific factors.

- *Accountability*—This indicates that the health-care providers, backed by the organization, own patient injury, and don't consider such injury as a threat. Rather, it creates a way to learn, so such injuries don't happen again.
- *Honesty*—The core of the UMHS is that of honesty, which focuses on rigorous self-evaluation of the method, process, and reasonableness of the care.
- *Principles*—This requires adherence to the model's three central principles of compensation, analysis of reasonable care, and reduction of patient injuries.
- *Dismissing fear*—This means getting rid of ligitation fears of disclosure among providers, of what might happen when honesty is in place.

In addition, UMHS, in the early going, intiated an online incident reporting system. This made it easier for patients to report injuries, thereby leading to early notification and an increase in potential claims (Boothman, Blackwell, Campbell Jr., Commiskey, and Anderson, 2009). As a note, an increase in claims is positive, as is an increase in compensation, so long as it is in tandem with a decrease in malpractice suits.

Furthermore, the UMHS CRP has made an effort to distinguish between reasonable and unreasonable care; in doing this, UMHS was able to develop methods to accomplish detailed investigations and expert assessments to understand the difference. Ultimately, the goal here has been to align both the interest of patients and UMHS by providing honest answers to questions raised by the patient's adverse outcome.

The question here, however, is did the UMHS model work? Research and information was gathered throughout the 2000s on the effect of the plan. In 2009, Boothman and colleagues pointed out that, unlike the dire predictions that indicated that "opening the door to medical errors would tap the previously untapped reservoir of claims" (see also Studdert, Mello, Gawande, Brennan, and Wang, 2007), UMHS actually saw the number of new claims fall, as shown in the following chart.

| Year | Number of Claims |
|---|---|
| 1999 | 136 |
| 2000 | 122 |
| 2001 | 121 |
| 2002 | 88 |

| 2003 | 81 |
| 2004 | 91 |
| 2005 | 85 |
| 2006 | 81 |

Also, during the time span of August 2001 to August 2007, the average claims processing time fell from 20.3 months to eight months, while total insurance reserves fell by more than two-thirds (Boothman, Imhoff, and Campbell Jr., 2012) and, just as important, were more than halved during this period of time. What is not known, however, is what the trend is today—the research only goes through 2010. However, the early research showed positive responses, proving that up-front disclosure and reasonable compensation could go a long way toward reducing lawsuits and costly litigation.

Finally, even as Boothman and his colleagues acknowledged that the program and its techniques pointed to an overall decrease in medical malpractice suits and reduced claim times and number of claims, the researchers also acknowledged that "surveys suggest that the UMHS approach may have achieved the unthinkable: It appears to satisfy doctors AND trial lawyers." Not only were patients satisfied, it seems, but both the medical and legal profession also ended up regarding this CRP in a positive light.

### ◆ University of Illinois at Chicago

In 2001, many regions across the United States experienced increasing medical malpractice premiums and large award judgments issued by juries (Lambert, et al., 2016). This, in turn, led malpractice insurance carriers to exit various markets, which then placed additional upward pressure on malpractice premiums (Lambert, et al., 2016; see also Freudenheim, 2001). It began costing more money for health-care organizations to obtain insurance policies, which were necessary in the face of increasing lawsuits and litigation.

The University of Illinois Medical Center of Chicago (UMCC), a 450-bed, academic-affiliated tertiery care center in Cook County, Illinois, was not immune to this issue of increased legal costs and rising malpractice insurance premiums. Furthermore, silence in the face of adverse medical events seemed to be the rule, rather than the exception. In fact, after two cases of serious medical errors that directly affected patients, hospital staff wanted to apologize to patients' families. They were, however, told by leadership not to do so, for fear of being killed in the media and for not having a specific process in place for apologies.

As this scenario was clearly untenable, for the staff, the patients, and the costs, the chief medical officer was charged with adapting a different approach for managing the health-care system's patient safety, medical liability, and risk profile. Taking a page from the University of Michigan's model, UMCC adapted its own CRP, known as a communication and optimal resolution program—CANDOR, for short—complete with a seven-pillar process. The process is deployed in the event of a patient harm event and focuses on the following:

1) incident reporting
2) investigation, while holding hospital bills and professional fees

3) early communication with the patient or family
4) full disclosure, apology, and rapid remedy, if needed
5) system improvement
6) data tracking and evaluation
7) education and training (Lambert, et al., 2016; see also McDonald et al., 2010)

The idea behind the seven pillars was that early and consistent communication with patients and families following an adverse medical event would build and maintain trust between the patient and health-care system, while leading to improved learning and reduced medical liability among the staff (Hickson and Entman, 2008). The program was put into place in hopes of reducing potential lawsuits, as well as reducing insurance premiums.

The early results from the program showed that there was no increase in lawsuits following implementation of the Seven Pillars program. There was also no increase in payouts from the self-insurance fund, which was related to full disclosure (McDonald, et al., 2010). As time went on, claims became less common, while settlement costs and legal fees also decreased. Additionally, annual contributions to the hospital's self-insurance fund declined dramatically; the fund moved from a $30 million deficit to a $40 million surplus.

Postresearch did find that the rate of lawsuits per claim decreased after implementation of the plan. There was, however, a brief postimplementation *increase* in lawsuits per claim, immediately following implementation of the program. Lambert et al. surmised that the reason was because the program initially was "more effective at preventing claims than preventing lawsuits." Eventually, the incidence of lawsuits did decrease; however, over the long-term, a focus on transparency in the face of medical error ended up costing less money.

While applauding the program (and similar CANDOR programs) for their effectiveness and cost reductions, McDonald et al. also cautioned that putting in a Seven Pillars or any other CANDOR type of program requires "significant institutional investment in risk management and an organisational commitment to provide swift peer review support when called into action." The problem is with institutions and organizations that are still steeped in a deny-and-defend mode, believing that early disclosure will automatically open the floodgates for malpratice lawsuits.

Still, the UICC study did demonstrate that, with implementation of a well-thought-out disclosure program, liabilities and payouts were significantly less than what might have otherwise happened.

## ◆ COPIC

In 2000, the COPIC Insurance Co., covering more than 80 percent of privately insured physicians in Colorado, launched a 3R program of disclosure (Kaiser, 2006). The 3Rs stand for recognize, respond, and resolve unanticipated medical outcomes, especially when it comes to medical errors. The program's purpose is to facilitate candid and early communication between health-care providers and their patients, in an effort to mitigate issues from adverse medical scenarios. Under the program, COPIC pays patients who have filed reasonable claims in the face of adverse medical events up to $25,000 for immediate medical expenses and up to $5,000 for lost time. While current metrics for this particular program were not available, as of 2005, the company had approximately 1,500 documented discussions concerning adverse events; out of those, 1,000 went no further, with 420 cases resulting in payments from $55 to $30,000. Thirty cases went into the claims department, and out of those thirty, nearly half closed, with no payment at all.

COPIC is an insurance company as opposed to a health-care organization. However, its program encourages early disclosure with an eye toward decreasing litigation. It seems as though when doctors and patients actually communicate with each other, costs involved with medical errors can decrease.

### ◆ Additional Research

As to the concern, which is often voiced, that immediate disclosure will give patients and their families ammunition to use against clinicians and hospitals if a matter should go to trial, research is proving that this isn't necessarily the case.

In addition to the aforementioned case studies, other research has been conducted to determine how CRPs affect the potential of malpractice litigation. One such study, which examined four Massachusetts hospitals, examined claims volumes, cost, and time to resolution before and after implementing a communication-and-resolution program (Kachala, et al., 2018). The researchers, in comparing that data to trends among nonimplementing institutions, found an improved success rate of new claims and a decline in legal defense costs at some hospitals. While the researchers indicated that the CRP didn't "significantly alter trends in other outcomes," they did allow that "none of the hospitals experienced worsening liability trends after CRP implementation," leading them to suggest that apology, transparency, and proactive compensation can be put into action without serious adverse financial consequences. Specifically, the fear that disclosure programs would automatically lead to a plethora of lawsuits, with medical centers buried under legal costs, has been, for the most part, unchallenged and proven to be untrue.

### ◆ Successes and Challenges

I say malpractice suits "can" be reduced through disclosure and communication programs, not necessarily "will be." While studies and overviews are starting to prove that apologies, through disclosures, when handled correctly, can go a long way toward reducing litigation, other scholars and researchers raise notes of caution on this topic. Waite (2005), for example, points out that "unrealistic expectations" shouldn't be raised with the idea that apologies and disclosure will automatically prevent litigation. "There will remain many cases where patients and families of victims will pursue litigation in any event," he noted, mainly to recover economic losses or to ensure that money becomes available for future care. Others might sue simply because they aren't satisfied with a given explanation or because no individuals were punished or held personally accountable. In other words, these plaintiffs or claimants might be out for revenge, with a lawsuit, by way of their thinking, possibly helping to assuage grief and bring closure. Still, while CANDOR programs or CRPs won't wipe out potential malpractice suits, Waite noted that this shouldn't get in the way of error disclosure programs or processes and apologies to patients for making a mistake.

One study observed six of the "early adaptors" of the CRP model to determine the challenges and successes of this method of dealing with adverse medical events. Two mentioned earlier, UMHS and UMCC, along with the Stanford University Medical Indemnity and Trust Insurance Company, were dubbed by researchers as "early settlement" programs or models when it came to disclosure and up-front honesty (Mello, et al., 2014). In other words, these programs investigated the standard of care in light of a particular adverse medical event, with no payout or compensation limits, including medical bill waivers and all economic losses suffered by the patient for his or her injury. Meanwhille, the COPIC Insurance Company, along with West Virginia Mutual Insurance Company and Conveys (formerly ProMutual Group), tends to follow limited-reimbursement models. Limited reimbursement does not investigate standard of care, though exclusion criteria does include death, notice of complaint, or written demand for payment, among other exclusions. Also, the compensation for the patient was capped at $30,000 (excluding medical bills), as well as out-of-pocket expenses or loss of time. Other differences as to the previous focused on the fact that the three early-settlement programs were developed in self-insured hospital systems, while the limited-reimbursement programs were developed by carriers not controlled by the facilities they insured. These institutions had different goals and methods in mind, which makes these two models reasonable for their particular purposes.

While most of the early disclosure programs did enjoy a share of success (as defined by declining malpractice claims and lawsuits), participants in both programs reported two major obstacles in developing and implementing the CRP plans, both of which involved the physicians and health-care providers.

### Practical Challenges

Educating the doctors was a challenge, not so much because they didn't grasp the concept, but because in many cases, physicians were situated at many different sites, in different states, at different practices, and with different insurance agents. The issue here was geographical; attempting to communicate with, and educate, physicians in different time zones and cities was difficult, especially without a coordinated effort. Effectively marketing the CRP to clinicians and physicians was crucial to ensuring its success, but not all received the same education at the same time. This meant that the learning curve involved with such programs ended up being fairly steep, and it took much longer for them to take hold.

### Lack of Buy-In

To say that the physicians were skeptical was an understatement. Mostly operating in the deny-and-defend, nondisclosure-at-all-costs culture of health care, many of the doctors weren't comfortable when it came to suddenly being asked to disclose mistakes to patients. The reluctance was likely due to a lack of training in that scenario and, as mentioned earlier, a "cultural disinclination to admit error." Also, as mentioned earlier, the health-care providers shared concerns that disclosure and settlement offers would lead to an increased liability risk, with the disclosure potentially being used in the event of a lawsuit. In this case, the focus was shifted from a legal risk and concerns to doing the right thing, but it still left many of the physicians involved concerned over the potential consequences.

## Concerns about Reporting

In addition to fearing legal reprisal when it came to disclosure, doctors were also concerned that participation in an early-disclosure program would end up triggering reports about them to state regulators or the National Practitioner Data Bank. Specifically, whenever a payout because of a medical error is made, the NPDB must be notified as to cause and amount. Reports to the National Practioner Data Bank are especially troubling from a physician's point of view, because once something is reported to the data bank, it's never removed. That information can be taken out and used against the physician in a future claim or lawsuit. Furthermore, negative reporting to the NPDB could led to problems when it comes to reputation or credentialing. In an effort to quell the fears of physicians, administrators with the limited-reimbursement CRPs assured the physicians that payments made through the program weren't required to be reported to federal and state authorities. Meanwhile, administrators of the early settlement programs developed a compromise, indicating they would report payments made in response to an adverse situation only in cases in which the physician, rather than the system, was the cause of the error.

Other challenges involved with these programs included ensuring timely incident reporting and the ability to conduct thorough and rapid investigations. In addition, managing patients' expectations was key; the participants in all six programs indicated it was a challenge to prevent patients and their families from having unrealistically high expectations for compensation.

In addition, the success of the programs were mainly attributed to what were called the "institutional champions," which ranged from senior administrators to the front-line staff administrators. Clinical leaders and respected physicians also served as program champions at some of the sites. This makes sense; when it comes to any kind of change management program, it's essential that champions be in place to drive the change and effort and support it. Without those leaders or champions supporting the program, it is likely to be doomed before it can even get off the ground.

A culture of transparency, it was revealed, was also essential to success—effective resolution of unanticipated care outcomes would be difficult to handle, unless people knew about it. In some cases, the hospital had a strong culture of transparency; among others, the culture of early reporting had to be built. I've mentioned deny-and-defend often enough in this book; attempting to build a successful disclosure program within a culture of denial is difficult without champions or some kind of incentive. In this case, incentives used to ensure early reporting and up-front disclosure included claims-made insurance policies. In other words, to trigger insurance coverage, providers with those policies needed to notify the insurer of any unantipcated care outcome or claim filed by a patient or his or her family during the policy period.

### ◆ Effectiveness and Rollout

While the CRP and CANDOR models have been effective, to an extent, with reducing malpractice claims and payouts, the question that needs to be asked is if such models can be adapted to a wide variety of health-care systems?

The Mello study of 2014 suggested the following lessons to be considered for organizations interested in implementing CRP programs.

*Understand that implementation of early disclosure programs is an investment.* Implementing the system and ensuring that it is successfully maintained require energy, political capital, and resources (financial and human). Buy-in from institutional leaders and other champions is absolutely critical for success. Speaking of which …

*A strong champion is a must.* One or more champions committed to the program are necessary to ensure that others will buy in. The enthusiasm of these champions will help bring other individuals on board, leading to a critical mass of acceptance.

*Understand the organization and its culture.* In the preceding examples, the University of Michigan had a culture different from that of the University of Illinois at Chicago. Furthermore, COPIC Insurance had different goals from the two university health-care systems. As such, strategic choices about the CRP designs need to be based on the organization's culture, structure, and needs. Mello and her colleagues pointed out that, for example, limited-reimbursement programs might be an easier sell in high risk-averse organizations, especially those in which physicians might be balking at the idea of early disclosure and compensation. However, both types of programs can be successfully operated in a variety of organizational structures.

*Don't be deterred by the legal and regulatory environment.* The interviewees in the Mello study indicated that, while damage caps and apology laws are helpful, they aren't essential to the success of an early disclosure program. In fact, in some cases, such legislation can actually hurt the effort. All leaders questioned by Mello and her colleagues did, however, emphasize the necessity of working with the state insurance departments and boards of licensing on an appropriate program design, to ensure that reporting requirements are triggered as seldom as possible.

*Overall, be patient.* The participants in the study were adamant that implementing a CANDOR program or CRP is not a quick fix that should be expected to fix things overnight. Rather, it takes time to implement this type of a program and to ensure it is effective. Developing and implementing a CRP requires a gradual cultural shift, with returns on investment not immediate but made over several years. Sometimes, a lack of immediate return on investment can deter even the most ardent supporter of a program. Again, returning to the idea of change management, it can take years for the process to sink in, and there will be setbacks as the organization struggles to change from its old ways into a new method of doing things. As such, organizations should be patient when it comes to implementing, and maintaining, an early disclosure program.

What is happening here is that programs are being developed to aid in early disclosure and compensation, in an attempt to reduce litigation (not to mention heartbreak and frustration from the patient).

However, the problem with some of these programs is that they don't include an apology as part of the process. While disclosure and "owning up" to medical error or adverse events is important—and the preceding are steps in the right direction—a disclosure program without acknowledgment of wrongdoing goes only so far. While a patient or patient's family might end up with some satisfaction from such a process, an expression of remorse is also important. Certainly, disclosure can help reduce the chances of litigation. But a proper apology (the result of an apology training program that teaches health-care providers the right way to say "I'm sorry"), issued on top of disclosure, can help bring emotional closure to both the perpetrator of the mistake (the physician / health-care provider) and the party who has been wronged (patient / patient's family).

### ◆ The Disclosure Process

While confession is certainly good for the soul, confessing wrongly might not be the best way to avoid litigation. Even the most honest health-care provider could find him- or herself in hot water, or in a courtroom, if involved with a poorly conducted disclosure discussion. For example, the physician or hospital representative needs to be careful of thoughtless or "flip" comments while talking to a patient or patient's family. Such comments could be misconstrued by an emotional patient as fact. For example, if a health-care provider makes a poor joke about "I know I didn't leave a gauze pad in a patient" to a patient's family following a surgery and then that patient either dies or is disabled in the wake of it, that "funny" comment could be taken as evidence of wrongdoing. As such, physicians do need to be careful when interacting with patients and their families and be aware that anything that is said, even as a joke, could be fodder in the event of a future lawsuit or litigation.

### ◆ All Disclosure, All the Time

The question we need to ask here, however, is how much is too much? Is it necessary to disclose nonharmful medical errors and near-misses, especially if no harm is done, and the patient isn't affected in a negative way? As we saw earlier, the medical ethicists are heartily in favor of all disclosure, all the time, pointing out that it is a physician's duty and obligation to disclose medical errors, even those that are not apparent, to patients. However, it can seem, from the health-care provider's point of view, that the idea of "no harm done" might be tempting in such a scenario; in other words, if a mistake doesn't have obvious consequences, then disclosure shouldn't be an issue. It simply doesn't need to be done.

The problem, however, is that certain mistakes and nondisclosures can have a tendency to come back up and hurt the physician or the organization. Having said that, there is no black and white when it comes to types of errors and their impact on patients. Misplacing a gauze pad, which, in turn, delays a change of bandage for a patient isn't necessarily fodder for disclosure (unless the delay can create serious injury, harm, or even death). A simple "I'm sorry this kept you waiting" from the nurse (who must also mean it) is likely going to be sufficient when it comes to preventing any problems. Furthermore, a patient isn't going to sue over a misplaced gauze pad, unless it means he or she is likely to bleed out. But keeping other incidents quiet isn't the way to go, either. Context is needed here, as is the degree of the error.

Chamberlain et al. (2012) indicate that yes, reporting of these incidents affects the patient-physician relationship in a positive way, while providing benefits to the medical system, as a whole. They assure the patient and family that the health-care provider and organization are doing their best to ensure effective health-care delivery. Furthermore, such reporting can help those in the organization understand that nonharmful medical errors are also potentially avoidable (Chamberlain, Koniarus, Wu, and Pawlik, 2012). Understanding the cause of such errors can help prevent future similar situations, which could eventually cause injury. Additionally, when it comes to medical error apologies, it's already been said that patients and their families want assurances that such errors won't occur again.

As such, even if the error in question didn't create any, or even lasting, harm, it's a good idea to have in place a system that allows reporting of such scenarios. It's also a very good idea to ensure that practitioners are trained in the art of apologizing.

# APOLOGIZING AND LITIGATION

**CAN APOLOGIZING STAND IN THE WAY OF LITIGATION?** Can it prevent a patient from calling his or her lawyer in the case of a medical error? There is little doubt that, in general, the act of apology can work wonders. We are human; when a situation caused by another person goes wrong, saying, "I'm sorry," can go a long way toward fixing the situation or at least to assuring the party who has been wronged that we are sincerely remorseful for what has happened, whether the fault for the mistake was ours or not.

In an earlier section in this book, I wrote extensively about the concept of "I'm sorry" and why, sometimes, that statement is necessary in the situation of an adverse medical event. Also, in that section, I wrote about apologies and apologizing in general terms and their effectiveness (or lack thereof) in making things better or satisfying the individual who was wronged. From an emotional standpoint, "I'm sorry," if properly delivered, shows empathy and remorse—many times, such an acknowledgment generates forgiveness from the party who has been wronged. This is the important aspect of an apology; the party perpetrating the wrong issues a heartfelt apology, allowing the party who has been wronged to begin the process of forgiveness. This give-and-take is important when it comes to developing emotional closure in such a situation. This also is effective if a physician makes a mistake during the process of medical treatment.

However, as I also mentioned in the preceding section, a physician who simply mouths the words in response to a mistake or adverse event isn't likely to obtain the necessary response, which would be forgiveness.

In this section, I'll apply the apology information written earlier to physicians and organizational early-disclosure programs. While apologizing can begin the process of forgiveness, simply apologizing can't be done in a vacuum. A proper apology, in conjunction with disclosure, is the way to help ensure that that the risk of litigation from a patient or patient's family is reduced.

### ◆ What Wronged Patients Need

It's been said throughout this book, when a medical error takes place, what patients want, in response, is fairly simple.

First, they expect an acknowledgment of wrongdoing. Patients (and their families) want to be sure that those responsible for making the mistakes understand the harm that was caused from the action, even if that action was unwitting. Patients and their families want the physician or health-care provider to own the error and to take responsibility for what happened. Patients don't necessarily want the physician in question to sink into a "mea culpa" abyss, but they do want acknowledgment that the error took place and the physician is aware of it and is taking responsibility for it (Leape, 2012). When her newborn son died from a medical error, Beth Daley Ullem was very clear in what, exactly, she wanted. She wanted someone to stand up and take responsibility for what happened. The fact that no one did so led her to the path of litigation.

Second, patients want an explanation as to what went wrong and why it went wrong. They want that explanation to be clear and concise—and above all, patients don't want to be talked down to. Many times, outlining the process that led to the error in question can help a patient understand the risks involved with the treatment. If, for example, corrective heart surgery went awry, with a patient's death as a result, telling the family, in detail, what happened, can help alleviate the trauma of loss. This is highly preferable to telling the family that "bad things happen," which can actually exacerbate a situation of loss.

Third, injured patients and their families expect an inquiry into why the mistake happened in the first place. They want the assurance that such a mistake will not happen again—and to be told about what is happening. "Knowing that another person is less likely to suffer in the same way gives positive meaning to an otherwise bad experience," Leape points out. Getting back to the example of our heart patient, the family might want to know that risks of such a surgery will be more explicitly outlined up front, especially if the patient is high-risk to begin with. They also might want to know that, perhaps, the amount of anesthesia used will be changed.

And the patient or family wants an apology—not just any apology but one that shows remorse, empathy, and an understanding that the mistake affected the physician as much as it's affecting the victim of the mistake. The family of the patient who died from the heart procedure wants to know that the surgeon empathizes with the situation and that everything possible to save the patient's life was done. Unlike what is assumed in a deny-and-defend culture, patients and families are, understandably, pretty forgiving when it comes to medical mistakes. When it comes to the heart patient, the family understood the risks, going in, as did the patient. Said Leape, "Patients don't expect perfect care and they understand that everything that occurs in a hospital is not under the control of their physician." What they do expect, Leape continued, is that their care is being overseen and that both the good and bad of the situation are being adequately addressed. In the example of the heart patient, it might be a good idea to remind the patient's family that, for example, the patient's high-risk profile included diabetes and kidney function problems as well as heart issues. Not that this makes up for the patient's death, but it can add clarity and information as to why that death should have been more expected. This isn't an apology, necessarily, but it does fall under the umbrella of "disclosure," also an important factor.

What's interesting about this particular list is that "compensation" isn't mentioned as a "must have" for acknowledging medical error. Certainly, patients might want to be compensated for medical bills or any extra pain and suffering that comes from an adverse medical event. And, as mentioned earlier, there could be patients or families who are out for revenge because they feel they're being wronged. The best way to obtain that revenge, they might be thinking, is to subject the physician or hospital where the mistake took place to a long, drawn-out litigation process. And there are others who are looking for a large payout and don't understand that the legal system doesn't really work that way.

But for the most part, obtaining million-dollar jury awards is not the sole aim of patients—or their families—who might be suffering from the result of an adverse event. Rather, the wronged parties want to know that the physician and health-care organization for which he or she works is aware of the problem, understands it, and will fix it. They also want to know that everything was done, during the process, to fix the problem or mistake, though the end result was, unfortunately, harm. And these parties want to be on the receiving end of an expression of remorse and empathy.

Though early-disclosure programs are proving to be very good for reducing claims and malpractice lawsuits, we can say that simply disclosing an error isn't enough. The patient in question wants an apology and an acknowledgment of the suffering that results from that error (Leape, 2012).

### ◆ Steps of an Effective Apology

With the preceding in mind, crafting and passing along an effective apology should be fairly straightforward. Leape (2012), for example, points out that the right apology "conveys respect, mutual suffering, and responsibility." Meaningful apologies, on the part of a patient's physician (and the institution for which he or she works), require responsibility, a show of remorse, and an offer to make amends (which would likely be in the hands of the organization in question). Leape also notes that, while the physician is required to play a lead role, it is up to the hospital to acknowledge the mishap, to take responsibility for ensuring it doesn't happen in the future, and to compensate for the error. Furthermore, the responsibility for ensuring this will all take place is in the hands of the hospital's CEO. In other words, the worst thing the hospital or health-care organization can do is to throw the erring physician under the bus, in an attempt to shift blame. As has been mentioned in this book, medical error, quite often, is the result of many interlocking activities and systems and the breakdown in one of those systems.

But meaningful apologies don't just happen. It's easy to say, "I'm sorry." Most of us do this on a daily basis, many times, reflexively, without true meaning to the words. It's also easy for a busy physician to say, "I'm sorry," thinking that will be enough and then to move on to the next case or patient. This apology to appease has no real emotion behind it, meaning the patient (and family) is left hanging, convinced that the physician doesn't care about his or her pain. If that patient is in emotional pain, as well, from the mistake that was made, he or she might decide taking revenge is the best path, with revenge taking the form of a lawsuit. This is why it's better not to apologize unless and until the physician is trained to make the right type of apology.

To that end, the health-care system or hospital needs to have policies and practices in place to ensure that every injured patient "is treated the way we would want to be treated ourselves—openly, honestly, with compassion and, when indicted, with apology and compensation." However, it is not necessarily easy for physicians or other health-care providers to make the right kind of apology. This is because issuing an apology that takes into account empathy and remorse requires training as to how this can be done. While some health-care providers (and some people, for that matter), are able to empathize instinctively, many others are not. A busy physician is not a bad person because he or she doesn't empathize. He or she is simply busy, with an extreme caseload. If this physician made a mistake, he or she is not likely to beat him- or herself over the head about it. This physician wants to apologize and to move on. This isn't his or her fault. Rather, he or she doesn't have the training or skills necessary to make the right apology. Nor does he or she have the time—physicians often have heavy caseloads. Their first priority is not necessarily going to be learning how to apologize correctly. However, it needs to be impressed upon the physician that a great deal is at stake in learning how to apologize.

Sociologist Nicholas Tavuchis (1991) opines an apology needs to be authentic and include the following:

1) acknowledging, through speech, the legitimacy of a violated rule
2) admitting fault for its violation
3) expressing genuine remorse and regret for harm caused by the violation

The operative word here, Tavuchis continued, was that, above all, an authentic apology should demonstrate *sorrow*.

To that end, training for physicians needs to be increased, while hospitals need to develop support programs for patients and caregivers. These hospitals also need to have support systems in place for physicians who have made errors. It takes more than apologizing to make the situation come out all right. Physicians need to be assured that they are still good people and good practitioners.

The basics of how, and when, to apologize are as follows.

*As soon as possible, following the event*

The truth here is that the longer someone waits to own up, the worse the damage. Turning to nonmedical examples, we've all seen what happens when a corporation makes a mistake and then doesn't own up to it immediately (but only does so when public pressure forces it to). The problem is compounded, stakeholders are angry, and the mistake and its ramifications are still apparent. The same thing happens with a medical error. The longer it takes to be acknowledged and apologized for, the more frustrated the patient will become. If that frustration remains and grows, it could lead to litigation.

*As part of a normal discourse with a patient or family*

In other words, simply coming out and saying, "I'm sorry I killed your husband while operating on him!" isn't the right way for a surgeon to admit error to a patient's family. This could be conceived of as an overemotional response; while it is an apology, it wouldn't exactly restore a family's faith that the husband/father received the right medical care. Rather, the surgeon should ensure that the family understands everything that happened in the operating room that led to the death. The family should be told that everything was done to save the patient's life, but ultimately, the patient died. And the surgeon should, if appropriate, inform the family as to his or her role in the mistake made. Finally, an appropriate apology should be given to the family. An ideal apology should invite open communication, offer empathy, and incorporate the "three Cs" of compassion, commitment, and any concerns. Such an apology should also allow the patient or family to vent, as well.

Can physicians and health-care providers be trained to make the "right kind" of apologies? The answer here is yes—but it takes a great deal of work and a great deal of buy-in by both physicians and the organizations for which they work. For the apology to be effective, physicians need to know how to say, "I'm sorry," and the health-care system needs to back that individual up. Furthermore, apology laws, in attempting to legislate sorry, also don't provide training to health-care providers on when, or how, to apologize (McMichael and Van Horn, 2019). Without proper training, in fact, apologies might be offered that actually increase malpractice liability risk. This is because most people can see through an insincere apology, meaning such an apology could create more harm than good.

For example, some doctors might apologize prematurely for an adverse event, in other words, before all the facts have been collected or validated. This can happen as part of a reflex action, one that is done without thinking. Apologizing in such situations could raise, in some patients' minds, the idea that there might have been a mistake in care. This could be a reflex apology, an apology issued because of a situational discomfort. The patient might not have realized that anything was wrong, but if a doctor or nurse comes into a room and blurts out wrongdoing, this could raise concerns about the level of care. This explains why apology laws might cause more harm than good—they simply mandate that physicians and organizations apologize, but they don't provide information about when or how to apologize. Typically, the best setting for any kind of apology is an open, rather than defensive, culture, in which health-care providers point out how the odds of a similar error will decrease—this is something that apology laws don't address. Basically, before apologizing for any kind of adverse medical event, the physician needs to understand what, exactly, went wrong and why (Taft, 2005). The same holds true when it comes to supporting a colleague's mistake. Sometimes, when we're working in a partnership with someone else and that individual makes a mistake, we might feel as though it is our responsibility as well. In response, we apologize, not only for ourselves, but for the partner who might have wronged the other individual. The problem with this is it isn't our responsibility to apologize. Doing so, without all the facts at hand, could create more problems than it solves. The same is true for physician error, especially if that error is the result of a colleague's actions. One physician apologizing for another's errors throws that other physician under the bus, which could potentially create tension within a partnership, as well as give the patient the wrong idea of what actualy occurred. As such, before apologizing on behalf of the colleague, the physician or health-care provider needs to have all the facts and an understanding as to what has taken place. This requires sitting down with a colleague and getting all the facts straight before issuing an apology (based on organizational requirements) to the wronged party.

This is also true when it comes to errors made by fellow clinicians or health-care providers. Gallagher et al. (2013) point out that patients and families must come first. However, before initiating a disclosure conversation about a colleague's potential error, it's important to get the facts—speculative or inaccurate information won't help matters. What is the best-case scenario is to initiate a colleague-to-colleague discussion about what happened; note Gallagher et al., "Interaction directly with the involved colleague is part of our professional responsibility."

## ◆ Empathy

Delving further into this concept, empathy, from a physician or health-care provider standpoint, is defined as that provider's ability to experience and share in a patient's feelings, the provider's intellectual ability to understand and identify another's feelings and perspective objectively and foster a communicative response to convey understanding of another (Roberts, 2007). The concept of empathy is also important when it comes both to disclosing medical error and apologizing for it (Hannan, et al., 2019). As I've been suggesting throughout this book, paying lip service to an apology doesn't really do much to make the patient feel better, nor does it help lessen the pain that patient feels. Basically, a provider who relates to a patient in a negative manner (being perceived as cold, less caring, or unfriendly) does face a higher risk of malpractice claims, than a provider who is perceived to relate to a patient in a positive manner (Hannan, et al., 2019; see also Shapiro et al., 1989). Specifically, health-care providers who are perceived as kinder, friendlier, and more caring have a less negative impact on a patient's perception of an adverse medical event. This, in turn, means a patient might be less likely to sue in the face of a medical mistake Now, not all people have empathy as part of their makeup, nor are they able to necessarily be empathetic on demand. As such, it's suggested that the need to teach empathy as part of a medical errors prevention program should be considered.

After determining that an apology should be made, the provider needs to make sure it's done well—a poorly done apology can make things worse (Roberts, 2007). A well-done apology involves at least four parts: acknowledgment, explanation, expression of remorse, and reparation (Roberts, 2007; see also Lazare, 2006). Other aspects essential for a well-thought-out apology should include who should be present (would the patients want other members of the family on hand?). Also, providers should be aware of their body language by mainaining an open and receptive posture and avoid jargon or defensive statements (Roberts, 2007). Above all, the provider needs to focus on listening and making sure the patient—and family—understands what has happened.

### ◆ Necessary Training

I've pointed out that not everyone knows how to apologize effectively. Expecting physicians to do so out of the blue is simply not realistic or fair to them. Such training can, and should, be started in medical school, which is also a good time to inform the budding doctors that they aren't God, and they will make mistakes. As such, rather than hiding behind the MD in an attempt to avoid the error, it's a better idea to acknowledge it and, when appropriate, express it.

One study focused on a pilot program among first-year medical students and helping to train them in the art of apologies and of apologizing correctly (Gillies, Speers, Young, and Fly, 2011). Gillies et al. point out in their study that training has typically focused on the experience of trainees in disclosing medical errors, involving traditional teaching interventions, such as readings, role plays, or case studies, with a small number of educational interventions relying on standardized procedures to teach disclosures. The problem, however, is that such methods offered limited practice opportunities, especially when it comes to real-world events. After all, apologizing to another student who is portraying an injured patient in a "role-playing" situation is vastly different from apologizing to an actual patient who has been injured as a result of a medical procedure or treatment.

Gillies and his colleagues, instead, developed an intervention for teaching medical students about medical errors and apologies, using Miller's clinical competence pyramid model, in which learners move from knowledge to competence to performance and action. Through the process, students were tasked with drafting an apology, analyzing the apology, analyzing how the apology made them feel, and then discussing the scenario with their peers and putting their apologies to a peer ranking. Furthermore, students were asked to adopt the patient's perspective when apologizing. The study had Gillies et al. suggesting methods in which external reviewers should analyze sample encounters between medical students admitting wrongdoing and their patients and then offer a specific review. However, other training modules advise residents only to discuss mistakes with patients rather than apologize (Peskin, 2018). Again, the apology is important in this scenario, as it can lead to potentially less litigation.

Finally, it's human nature to show remorse in the face of any adverse event. When a human being hurts another one, the first reaction is to want to make it better. And the first step to making things better is to apologize, with remorse.

Doctors are no different—if they know they are in the wrong (or that their organization is in the wrong), they want to acknowledge it and apologize for it. This goes back to the "forgiveness" aspect of an apology; once the practitioner apologizes and the patient (or the patient's family) forgives, then both parties can move on and leave the emotional episode behind them.

Studies are proving that physicians and health-care providers tend to suffer from anxiety when it comes to restrictions and concerns about what they are and are not allowed to discuss (Tan, 2016; see also Elwy, et al., 2016). In a deny-and-defend organizational culture, keeping silent is common, but this can hurt physicians and staff. One study focused on surgeons and disclosure of adverse events showed that the surgeons who were less likely to discuss preventability of the adverse events or who reported difficult communication experiences were more negatively affected by the ultimate disclosure when it took place. This proves the point that medical professionals need more than simply being told to apologize in the face of an adverse event. They also need training on how to properly do so.

### ◆ Involving the Patient

Furthermore, by not disclosing and apologizing, health-care organizations are wasting a potentially valuable resource when it comes to improving outcomes—namely, involving the patients. Sometimes patients themselves can end up being helpful when it comes to identifying adverse events and how and why they took place. They are, after all, the ones who have experienced the events and can discuss those events firsthand, especially if they are asked for their feedback and opinion on the event.

But why would the medical establishment want to query the family members of patients who have experienced some kind of adverse situation? Wouldn't there be negative feedback or pushback if the patients are questioned? Perhaps. But more often than not, the health-care organization itself might not even be aware of the error (Etchegaray, et al., 2016). Again, the patients are the ones who are on the receiving end of that care; many times, doctors, nurses, or clinicians might be too busy or too distracted to realize what is happening and what a patient is thinking or feeling on a physical basis. They might not realize, for example, that they are putting a blood pressure cuff on a sore arm—that is, unless, the patient speaks up.

To that end, health-care organizations, more and more, are starting to recognize that information obtained from the patient and family during the error dislosure process can be very useful for event analysis and possible prevention of recurrence (Zimmerman and Amory, 2017). It also tells the patient that his or her opinion or experience matters when it comes to error disclosure.

Another reason is because the patient him- or herself might be the only person who has seen or who understands that a communication breakdown has taken place between him- or herself and a provider (Etchegaray, et al., 2016). And many times, the families of patients are the single connecting thread of continuity between various providers and specialists who might otherwise not communicate with one another. When questioned correctly, therefore, the patients and their families can be a welcome resource to delving into the anatomy of a medical error. Furthermore, patients and their families want to feel included in the process, so asking them questions could be a very good step when it comes to understanding why a mistake took place. In this case, patients and families are "customers" of a hospital. In any other business, customer feedback is routinely solicited when it comes to product or service satisfaction. There is no reason why patients shouldn't be allowed the same participation or the same courtesy.

Noted Etchegaray et al., "When an organization fails to ask patients and family members about factors contributing to their event, potentially valuable information from them is lost, and not considerd in the event analysis" (p. 2601).

### ◆ Sorry Works! To an Extent

There have been programs put in place to help encourage healthcare organizations to implement apologies in the event of adverse events or medical error. In 2005, the Sorry Works! Coalition was launched, with the message that apologies for medical errors, combined with up-front compensation, can lead to a reduction in medical malpractice lawsuits and legal costs (Wojcieszak, Banja, and Houk, 2006; see also Sorry Works! (Our Approach), 2019). The coalition is made up of doctors, lawyers, insurers, and patient advocates dedicated to incorporating full disclosures and apologies as a "middle-ground" solution to medical mapractice. The coalition is also dedicated to overcoming cultural and legal barriers to full disclosure—the coalition points out that the medical profession itself is the greatest disclosure to apologizing and compensation. While the website and articles don't have specifics as to whether their system has a causal realationship with a drop in malpractice suits, they do introduce information about why apologizing is necessary—and how to craft an ideal apology that will at least make a patient think before he or she decides to contact a lawyer.

In fact, literature in recent years is showing that erosion of deny-and-defend is leading to some stellar results when it comes to doctor-patient relationships. When a physician apologizes for wrongdoing, a great weight is lifted from that individual's shoulders and the patient understands that the physician tried his or her best and was human and made a mistake. With an apology comes the acknowledgment of a mistake, as well as the understanding that the mistake will likely not happen again.

In the preceding comments, we mentioned David Hilfiker, who apologized to a patient for an error he made. In another scenario, Sharon O'Brien, MD, found herself in a dire situation when a medical error brought a patient into her ICU (Tan, 2016). The patient eventually died, and O'Brien was faced with what to tell the family and how to tell them that they had lost their loved one. After thinking about the scenario, she opted to be honest with the family and braced herself to face their anger, even though technically, the patient's death wasn't strictly her fault but rather, was the result of a medical error for which she wasn't responsible. To her surprise, rather than being angry, however, the grief-stricken family appreciated O'Brien's honesty and forthrightness. This is not to suggest that all families would be as sympathetic or supportive in similar situations—people are, after all, human and respond to grief and tragedy in different ways. However, the assumption that families are going to be angry and automatically sue when the truth is issued is patently false, as Dr. O'Brien found out.

The one problem she faced, however, was that while the family was supportive and appreciative of her honesty, O'Brien didn't receive the same support or respect from the hospital. Wile her decision helped the family, she acknowledged that "I felt so unsupported in that experience." This could be because the hospital for which she worked really didn't have a way for her to work through her own grief or guilt with the situation. As such, it's interesting to note that the hospital actually allowed O'Brien to apologize. As we've seen in this book, many other health-care organizations would have told her to keep her mouth shut and to say nothing. This, of course, is the wrong thing to do.

When implemented as part of a hospital or system-wide program, well-practiced apologies have been shown to reduce both the frequency and size of medical malpractice claims (McMichael, 2018). One well-documented apology program, which was outlined here, was implemented at the University of Michigan Health System. A study examining the program showed that, after implementation, the number of monthly claims focused on demands for compensation decreased by 36 percent, while the number of lawsuits fell by 65 percent, relative to the preimplementation rates (McMichael, 2018; see also Kachalia et al., 2010). In addition, of the claims and lawsuits that were filed, the hospital saved nearly 60 percent in compensation paid out to claimants, while seeing its mean lawsuit costs fall from more than $400,000 to just over $225,000. A later study of the Michigan program went further, finding that payments to claimants decreased by 47 percent, while time to resolution also decreased from nearly two years to six months (Adams, Elmunzer, and Scheiman, 2014). However, an apology program is only as good as the institution putting it into action—McMichael (2019) noted that a health-care system-specific apology program often requires "that institutions take affirmative actions to implement it, limiting its generalizability."

### ◆ Implementing Enterprise Risk Management

When it came to the discussion about early disclosure programs, such as CRP (and CANDOR, specifically), the emphasis was on organizational culture and the willingness of that culture to take on the program. Both preventing and disclosing medical errors requires specific organizational and systemic management strategies (Sorrell, 2017). This, in turn, requires organizational change.

When it comes to disclosure/apology programs in a health-care setting, practitioners and executives can take a page from the concept of enterprise risk management. An enterprise risk management (ERM) framework, especially in health care, can help organizational members to understand risk management and to make risk management decisions that offer value protection and creation by managing risk and uncertainty. The goal of an effective ERM is to reduce harm to stakeholders connected with a health-care organization, from the patients and their families to physicians and other health-care providers (ASHRM, 2019).

The concept of an ERM is that it encompasses the entire enterprise or organization. In other words, use of this tool when it comes to protecting against litigation needs to go beyond a single department and needs to take into account all aspects of organizational behavior. The framework also recognizes risk and takes action, ahead of time, to deal with that risk (ASHRM, 2019).

For example, there is absolutely no doubt that mistakes will happen in medical care, especially when it comes to high-risk surgeries. As such, ERM processes take into account that high-risk surgeries can end up causing injuries, or even death, just as often (if not more) than they can succeed. Through an ERM framework, all possible surgical outcomes are weighed, with responses along with them. If the surgery is a success, then the surgeon and his or her team can tell the family (and patient) the good news, while indicating potential postoperative risks (such as infections). If the surgery results in injury or death, however, the ERM provides responses that the surgeon can make to the family, which might include immediate disclosure, an expression of sincere remorse, and appropriate compensation, if it gets that far. The ERM prepares an organization for all events and scenarios, while putting into place appropriate responses and actions.

According to the American Society for Health Care Risk Management, an ERM system's guiding principles include the following building blocks (ASHRM, 2019):

- advance safe and trusted health care
- manage uncertainty
- maximize value protection and creation
- encourage multidisciplinary accountability
- optimize organizational readiness
- promote positive organizational culture

- utilize data and metrics with priorities risks
- align risk appetite and strategy

Furthermore, ERM practices are continuous and require a shift in how the organization identifies and recognizes risks and opportunities (ASHRM, 2019). Managing risk through enterprise risk management is an ongoing journey—in other words, continuous improvement is an important feature in this process.

Going further, the ERM risk domains cover everything from operational to techological to legal and regulatory issues. For our purposes, the "operational" and "clinical/patient safety" domains are important and are as follows (ASHRM, 2019):

### Operational

Operational risks are those that result from poor or inadequate internal processes, people, or systems that might affect business operations. This is where deny-and-defend comes in; if there are poor internal processes when it comes to harm from medical error, then the mistake is never acknowledged. It's hidden and could lead a patient or family to bring suit against the physician or organization. To avoid this potential from occuring, it's important that the organization move from a "circle the wagons" mentality into one that allows and encourages disclosure (trained disclosure), as well as a compensation setup, when warranted. Additionally, an ERM can alert other departments when an adverse medical event is taking place. For example, one issue that infuriated Beth Daley Ullem (and rightfully so) was that, in the midst of grieving for her newborn son and attempting to receive information about why he died, she kept being billed for her care, to the tune of $90,000. The lack of communication to the billing department was sad. If that hospital had had a viable ERM in place, it's likely the billing department would have been asked to place a "hold" on the bill, at least until the situation was resolved to everyone's satisfaction.

### *Clinical/Patient Safety*

This particular risk focuses on delivery of care to residents, patients, and other health-care stakeholders or customers. Such risks can include failure to follow evidence-based practices, medication errors, serious safety events, and hospital-acquired conditions (such as infections or falls). Putting into place a risk management program that takes into account the safety of patients is important. Even in the most streamlined and well-run organization, mistakes and errors of judgment will happen. The ERM framework helps leadership and risk managers weigh the likelihood of any type of potential risk and, once again, develop solutions to mitigate that risk. As an example, if postsurgical infection is considered a high-risk area, then risk management can focus on steps to ensure that such infection is minimized. These steps can include proper hygiene (hand-washing before touching or examining a patient), limiting family members postsurgery, encouraging visitors to wear masks when visitng the patient, and ensuring that the room in which a patient is recuperating is as sanitary and clean as possible. While it's difficult to avoid all health-care risks to a patient, the ERM helps an organization ensure that it can do everything it can to ensure a reduction of risk.

Furthermore, enterprise risk management is ideal for when it comes to disclosure and apologizing for a medical error in the following ways.

*It empowers practitioners.* One issue that physicians and other health-care providers face is lack of organizational support in the event of a medical error. An ERM helps ensure that practioners have that support, as the framework has already determined potential risks and solutions to meeting those risks. If a patient dies in the course of a particular treatment, the practitioner responsible for that patient already knows what to do. Erasing uncertainty from actions provides a "freeing" mentality, meaning the physician is under less stress from a potential "what if."

*It allows a more holistic viewpoint.* An effective ERM framework allows the organization to focus on potential issues and risks in a more "holistic" front, examining the positive and negative outcomes. Rather than focusing solely on a potentially negative outcome, the ERM assists in determining what could go wrong and then provides potential solutions to mitigate the risk.

*It helps provide a greater competitive benefit to truth telling.* The concept of deny-and-defend seems to involve the idea that there is no such thing as a mistake and that if a mistake happens, burying it is the best way to ensure that it goes away. The reality is, when a mistake happens, the consequences can be far-reaching, and no amount of denial will erase that fact. Beth Daley Ullem's newborn died from medical error. Ullem realized that no amount of denial or stonewalling would get rid of the cause (medical error) or the result (her baby's death). If, however, the hospital in question had worked from an enterprise resource management framework, the response to the death might not have been silence. Rather, it might have been disclosure and apology, because the hospital would have understood that sometimes bad things happen to patients, and the doctor would have been prepared for that bad thing to happen, and would have known how to respond to the situation. Or, what is more likely, is that an ERM might have caught the reasons why newborns were dying, through a systematic analysis of systems and processes. This leads us to the final point:

*An ERM process ensures examination of primary domains.* Because setting up an ERM framework involves examining risk and then putting into place solutions to mitigate that risk, the process involves an in-depth look at all departments and procedures. The analysis takes into account activities that can magnify risk and then provides solutions as to how to lessen it. It is impossible to eliminate all risk—no organization has the time or resources to do that. But it does ensure that leadership understands the potential of risk in a hospital's domains. With that understanding, responses and results can be developed. The overall goal in this situation is preparation.

Along with disclosure, admission of wrongdoing, and apologies, implementation of enterprise risk management can help a health-care organization handle fallout from a medical error or can even help mitigate that medical error in the first place. Unlike deny-and-defend, an ERM allows a health-care organization to examine processes and personnel with a clear-eyed, honest look; envision specific scenarios; and then come up with tools in an attempt to mitigate the risk of those scenarios. However, as with anything dealing with owning up to medical errors, development and implementing an ERM framework requires a systematic organizational shift. Organizational readiness is essential for ensuring that an ERM framework can be effective for both mitigating the risk of medical error and responding to it should it occur.

And again, organizational change is an important component of ERM. Without a meaningful change management process in place, much like apology programs or disclosure efforts, the risk management potential won't go anywhwere.

# DISCUSSION

It has been demonstrated in many studies that both doctors and patients believe that improved commnication between patients and physicians—especially in dealing with medical error—could reduce future malpractice litigation (Carroll, 2015). This delves into admitting wrongdoing in the event of a medical error.

The focus of this book was whether saying "I'm sorry" for an adverse medical event would be enough to head off potentially disastrous litigation for the physician or hospital. The point here was that yes, apologizing to a point can be a deterrent to litigation. Another point is that the current culture involved with health-care organizations that deny-and-defend isn't doing a very good job of preventing malpractice litigation from taking place. Because of this, other alternatives need to be investigated.

If an apology is crafted in the right way—in other words, it's well thought out rather than brusque or off the cuff—it can be a good start when it comes to making the victim (i.e., the patient or his or her family) feel less angry or frustrated with the situation. The issue with apologizing, however, is that it's difficult for many physicians to do. It is, in fact, difficult for many human beings to craft an adequate apology, one that conveys remorse, empathy, and a sincere desire to do better next time. Given that nonmedical people struggle with apologizing, it's a bit of a stretch to throw practitioners into a situation and expect them to nail the apology when it comes to making up for a medical error.

Because of this, the art of apology needs to be trained. A poor apology, in fact, can be worse than no apology at all; as such, a health-care system or hospital should have in place an apology training program. The physicians and other health-care providers need to be trained appropriately and supported when an error happens. This is because a physician can become involved in self-blame when something goes wrong, and keeping silent about it (or having the organization throw this person under the bus) is the worst thing that a hospital can do. Many nonmedical organizations are quick to forgive an errant employee when a mistake is made. It's unconscionable that physicians aren't forgiven by the organizations for which they work.

And in addition to apologizing, disclosure is an important aspect when it comes to heading off litigation. There is no support to the belief that disclosure or apologies lead to more litigation, which is what the deny-and-defend culture would have one believe. Rather, in this book, I proved, through research and anecdotal evidence, that patients want to get to the bottom of an adverse medical event; they want to know what went wrong, why it went wrong, and if the hospital or institution is going to do something about it. In fact, as was pointed out in the story that introduced this book, silence is the worst way to go about dealing with a medical error. If we accept the premise that patients and their families want information, then keeping quiet about a scenario isn't going to delay litigation—it will likely drive it. The lawyers advising health-care organizations won't support the idea of disclosure or apologizing, namely because it likely cuts into their billable hours. Risk managers don't like it either. The truth, however, is that a disclosure and apology program are important to let the patients and their families know that something wrong has taken place, that the health-care organization and practitioner are aware of the issue, that the issue is being dealt with, and that all involved are sorry and remorseful. Appropriate compensation is an added benefit to this process.

Also important is to ensure that the discussion is presented in such a way to minimize a colleague's defensiveness; in other words, an adverse medical event should be discussed in an open and honest manner, without a rush to judgment (Gallagher, et al., 2013). Finally, institutional leadership is just as important, especially when many health-care providers have been involved or communication between providers has broken down (Conway, Stewart, and Campbell, 2011). The institution should also ensure that a culture is in place in which individuals are encouraged to provide safety-related information and rewarded for doing so.

Regardless of the type of CRP involved with the process, it's important to shift a health-care organization's culture from one of deny-and-defend to one of openness and communication. Doing so is not a quick fix—there needs to be buy-in from all parties, as well as champions and leadership to ensure that this shift is conducted in an appropriate manner. It will take time. But shifting to this type of culture will ensure that litigation will fall, meaning legal and compensation costs should also decrease.

To conclude, the practice of medicine is dangerous. On a daily basis, practitioners are responsible for ensuring that people fight off diseases that once claimed lives. Babies are delivered from mothers; in the past, those mothers might have died from various postbirth complications. And on a daily basis, surgeons are opening our bodies or performing laser procedures on everything from relieving a sore back to transplanting a heart or lung. If we examine the practice of medicine in this context, it's a miracle that more mistakes don't occur. But the truth is that there is no such thing as "foolproof medicine." It's a risk. People will be injured during treatment (or from a lack of it). They will die. It's part of it.

Most patients are accepting of the fact that there is a risk to the practice of medicine. And while there are a few who are trigger-happy when it comes to litigation, most just want to be kept in the loop when something goes wrong. Disclosure of medical errors is a moral obligation; the physician is required, based on the reason why he or she opted to practice medicine, to let a patient and family know what's going on and when mistakes happen. Furthermore, a disclosure, combined with a well-crafted and heartfelt apology, goes a long way toward showing the physician that the practitioner is on his or her side and that this physician has the patient's best interests at heart.

# REFERENCES

Ackerman, B. G. (2018, November 6). "You Had Me at 'I'm Sorry': The Impact of Physicians' Apologies on Medical Malpractice Litigation." Retrieved from The National Law Review: https://www.natlawreview.com/article/you-had-me-i-m-sorry-impact-physicians-apologies-medical-malpractice-litigation.

Adams, M., Elmunzer, B., and Scheiman, J. (2014, April). "Effect of a Health System's Medical Error Disclosure Program on Gastroenterology-Related Claims Rates and Costs." *American Journal of Gastroenterology, 109*(4), 460–464. doi:10.1038/ajg.2013.375.

*AHA Patient's Bill of Rights.* (1992, October 21). Retrieved from American Patient Rights Association: https://www.americanpatient.org/aha-patients-bill-of-rights/.

AHRQ. (2016). *Communication and Optimal Resolution (CANDOR) Toolkit.* Retrieved from Agency for Healthcare Research and Quality: https://www.ahrq.gov/patient-safety/capacity/candor/modules.html.

Allan, A., and McKillop, D. (2010, April). "The Health Implications of Apologizing after an Adverse Event." *International Journal for*

*Quality in Health Care, 22*(2), 126–131. doi:doi.org/10.1093/intqhc/mzq001.

Anderson, N. (2017). "A Brief History of Medical Malpractice." Retrieved from Physician News Digest: https://physiciansnews.com/2017/05/10/brief-history-medical-malpractice/.

ASHRM. (2019, June). "Enterprise Risk Management." Retrieved from American Society for Health Care Risk Management: https://www.ashrm.org/system/files?file=media/file/2019/06/ERM-Tool_final.pdf.

Berdine, G. (2015, January). "The Hippocratic Oath and Principles of Medical Ethics." *The Southwest Respiratory and Critical Care Chronicles, 3*(9), 28–32. doi:10.12746/swrccc 2015.0309.115.

Berlinger, N. (2008). "Chapter 21—Medical Error." In E. Mary Crowley, *From Birth to Death and Bench to Clinic: The Hastings Center Bioethics Briefing Book for Journalists, Policymakers and Campaigns* (pp. 97–100). Garrion, NY: The Hastings Center.

Boodman, S. G. (2017, March 12). "Should Hospitals—and Doctors—Apologize for Medical Mistakes?" Retrieved from *Washington Post*: https://www.washingtonpost.com/national/health-science/should-hospitals--and-doctors--apologize-for-medical-mistakes/2017/03/10/1cad035a-fd20-11e6-8f41-ea6ed597e4ca_story.html.

Boothman, R. (2016, December). "CANDOR: The Antidote to Deny and Defend?" *Health Services Research, 51*, 2487–2490. doi:10.1111/1475-6773.12626.

Boothman, R., Blackwell, A., Campbell Jr., D., Commiskey, E., and Anderson, S. (2009, January). "A Better Approach to Medical

Malpractice Claims? The University of Michigan Experience." *Journal of Health Life and Science Law, 2*(2), 125–159.

Boothman, R. C., Imhoff, S. J., and Campbell Jr., D. A. (2012, Spring). "Nurturing a Culture of Patient Safety and Achieving Lower Malpractice Risk through Disclosure: Lessons Learned and Future Directions." *Frontiers of Health Services Management, 28*(3), 13–28.

Brennan, T. A., Leape, L. L., Laird, N. M., Heberg, L., Localio, R. A., Lawthers, A. G., … Hiatt, H. H. (1991). "Incidence of Adverse Events and Negligence in Hospitalized Patients: Results of the Harvard Medical Practice Study I." *New England Journal of Medicine*(324), 370–376. doi:10.1056/NEJM199102073240604.

Carroll, A. E. (2015, June 1). "To Be Sued Less, Doctors Should Consider Talking to Patients More." Retrieved from *New York Times*: https://www.nytimes.com/2015/06/02/upshot/to-be-sued-less-doctors-should-talk-to-patients-more.html.

Cauchi, R. (2018, December 17). "State Laws and Action Challenging Certain Health Reforms." Retrieved from National Conference of State Legislatures: http://www.ncsl.org/research/health/state-laws-and-actions-challenging-ppaca.aspx.

Chamberlain, C. J., Koniarus, L. G., Wu, A. W., and Pawlik, T. M. (2012, March). "Disclosure of "Nonharmful" Medical Efforts and Other Events." *Archives of Surgery, 147*(3), 282–286. doi:doi:10.1001/archsurg.2011.1005.

Cleopas, A., Villaveces, A., Charvet, A., Bovier, P., Kolly, V., and Perneger, T. (2006). "Patient Assessments of a Hypothetical Medical Error: Effectves of Health Outcome, Disclosure, and

Staff Responsiveness." *Quality and Safety in Health Care, 15*(2), 136–141.

*Code of Ethics of the American Medical Association*. (1847). Chicago, IL: American Medical Association.

Cohen-Almagor, R. (2017, December). "On the Philosophical Foundations of Medical Ethics: Aristotle, Kant, J. S. Mill and Rawls." *Ethics, Medicine and Public Health, 3*(4), 436–444. doi:10.1016/j.jemep.2017.09.009.

Conway, J., Stewart, K., and Campbell, M. (2011). *Respectful Management of Serious Clinical Adverse Events.* 2nd ed. IHI Innovation Series White Paper. Cambridge, MA: Institute for Healthcare Improvement.

Davidoff, F. (2002). "Shame: The Elephant in the Drawing Room." *Quality and Safety in Health Care, 11*, 2–3.

Donaldson, M. S. (2008). "An Overview of *To Err is Human*: Re-emphasizing the Message of Patient Safety." In E. Ronda G Hughes, *Patient Safety and Quality: An Evidenced-baseed Handbook for Nurses*. Rockville, MD: Agency for Healthcare Research and Quality.

Edwin, A. (2009, March). "Non-disclosure of Medical Errors: An Egregious Violation of Ethical Principles." *Ghana Medical Journal, 43*(1), 34–39.

Egan, E. (2004, March). "Patient Safety and Medical Error: A Constant Focus in Medical Ethics." *Virtual Mentor, Journal of Ethics of the American Medical Associationo, 6*(3), 101–102. doi:10.1001/virtualmentor.2004.6.3.fred1-0403.

Elwy, A., Itani, K., Bokhour, B., Mueller, N., Clickman, M., Zhao, S., ... Gallagher, T. (2016, November). "Surgeons' Disclosure of Clinical Adverse Events." *JAMA Surgery, 151*(11), 1015–1021. doi:https://www.ncbi.nlm.nih.gov/pubmed/27438083.

Etchegaray, J. M., Ottosen, M. J., Aigbe, A., Sedlock, E., Sage, W. M., Bell, S. K., ... Thomas, E. J. (2016, December). "Patients as Partners in Learning from Unexpected Events." *Health Services Research*, 2600–2614. doi:10.1111/1475-6773.

FindLaw. (2019). "Mediation vs. Arbitration vs. Litigation: What's the Difference?" Retrieved from FindLaw.com: https://adr.findlaw.com/mediation/mediation-vs-arbitration-vs-litigation-whats-the-difference.html.

Freudenheim, M. (2001, December 13). "St. Paul Cos. Exits Medical Malpractice Insurance." Retrieved from *New York Times*: https://www.nytimes.com/2001/12/13/business/st-paul-cos-exits-medical-malpractice-insurance.html.

Friedman, H. (2012, August-September). "Ten Days of Apologies." Retrieved from Jewish Magazine: http://www.jewishmag.com/168mag/ten_days_of_repentence/ten_days_of_repentence.htm.

Gallagher, T. H., Waterman, A. D., Ebers, A. G., Fraser, V. J., and Levinson, W. D. (2003, February 26). "Patients' and Physicians' Attitudes Regarding the Disclosure of Medical Errors." *JAMA—Journal of the American Medical Association, 289*(8), 1001–1007.

Gallagher, T., Barbutt, J. M., Waterman, A. D., Rlum, D. R., Larson, E. B., Waterman, B. M., ... Levinson, W. (2006, August 14). "Choosing Your Words Carefully: How Physicians Would Disclose Harmful Medical Errors to Patients." *Archivest of Internal Medicine, 166*(15), 1585–1593. doi:10.1001/archinte.166.15.1585.

Gallagher, T., Mello, M. M., Levinson, W., Wynia, M. K., Sachdeva, A. K., Sulmasy, L. S., … Arnold, R. (2013, October 31). "Talking with Patients about Other Clinicians' Errors." *New England Journal of Medicine, 369*(18), 1752–1757. doi:10.1056/NEJMsb1303119.

Gawande, A., Thomas, E., Zinner, M., and Brennan, T. (1999, July). "The Incidence and Nature of Surgical Adverse Events in Colorado and Utah in 1992." *Surgery, 126*(1), 66–75.

Ghazai, L., Saleem, Z., and Amlani, G. (2014). "A Medical Error: To Disclose or Not to Disclose." *Journal of Clinical Research & Bioethics, 5*(2), 174. doi:10.4172/2155-9627.1000174.

Gillies, R. A., Speers, S. H., Young, S. E., and Fly, C. A. (2011, June). "Teaching Medical Error Apologies: Development of a Multi-Component Intervention." *Family Medicine, 43*(6), 400–406.

Glaser, B. (1966, Summer). "Disclosure of Terminal Illness." *Journal of Health and Human Behavior, 7*(2), 83–91. doi:10.2307/2948723.

Goguen, D. (2019). "Negligence, the "Duty of Care," and Fault for an Accident." Retrieved from NOLO: https://www.nolo.com/legal-encyclopedia/negligence-the-duty-care-fault-accident.html.

Golan, D. (2011). "Dropped Medical Malpractice Claims: Their Surprising Frequency, Apparent Causes and Potential Remedies." *Health Affairs, 30*(7), 1343–1350.

Gorski, D. (2019, February 4). *Are medical errors really the third-most common cause of death in the U.S.?* Retrieved from Science-Based Medicine: https://sciencebasedmedicine.org/are-medical-errors-really-the-third-most-common-cause-of-death-in-the-u-s-2019-edition/.

Gorton, C. (2005, July-August). "Using Mediation to Resolve Disputes in Health Care." *Physician Executive*, pp. 34–37.

Grober, E. D., and Bohnen, J. M. (2005, February 2). "Defining Medical Error." *Canadian Journal of Surgery, 48*(1), 39.

Guthrie, D. J., Underwood, E. A., Richardson, R. G., Rhodes, P., and Thomson, W. A. (2019). *History of Medicine.* Retrieved from Britannica: https://www.britannica.com/science/history-of-medicine.

Hannan, J., Sanchez, G., Musser, E. C., Ward-Peterson, M., Azutillo, E., Goldin, D., ... Foster, A. (2019). "Role of Empathy in the Perception of Medical Errors in Patient Encounters: A Preliminary Study." *British Medical Journal Research Notes, 12*(327), 2–5. doi:10.1186/s13104-019-4365-2.

Harchol, H., and Kaye, L. (n.d.). "Repair and Apology: What Does Judaism Teach Us?" Retrieved from Reform Judaism: https://reformjudaism.org/repair-and-apology-what-does-judaism-teach-us.

Helo, S., and Moultaon, C.-A. E. (2017, August). "Complications: Acknowledging, Managing, and Coping with Human Error." *Transationa Andrology and Urology, 6*(4), 773–782. doi:10.21037/tau.2017.06.28.

Hickson, G., and Entman, S. (2008). "Physician Practice Behavior and Litigation Risk: Evidence and Opportunity." *Clinical Obstetrics & Gynecology, 51*(4), 688–699.

Hilfiker, D. (1984). "Facing Our Mistakes." *New England Journal of Medicine, 310,* 118–122. doi:10.1056/NEJM198401123100211.

Ho, B., & Liu, E. (2011). "Does Sorry Work? The Impact of Apology Laws on Medical Malpractice." *Journal of Risk & Uncertainty, 43,* 141.

Hyman, C., Liebman, C., Schechter, C., and Sage, W. (2010, October). "Interest-Based Mediation of Medical Practice Lawsuits: A Route to Improved Patient Safety?" *Journal of health Politics, Policy and Law,* 35(5), 797–828. doi:10.1215/03616878-2010-028.

Jackson, J. (2001). *Truth, Trust and Medicine.* New York, NY: Routledge.

Jenkins, R. C., Firestone, G., Aasheim, K. L., and Boelens, B. W. (2017, September). "Mandatory Pre-Suit Mediation for Medical Malpractice: Eight-Year Results and Future Innovations." *Conflict Resolution Quarterly,* 35(1), 73–88. doi:10.1002/crq.21194.

Kachala, A., Sands, K., Van Niel, M., Dodson, S., Roche, S., Novack, V., … Mello, M. M. (2018, November). "Effects of a Communication-and-Resolution Program on Hospitals' Malpractice Claims and Costs. *Health Affairs,* 37(11), 1836–1844. doi:10.1377/hlthaff.2018.0720.

Kachalia, A., Kaufman, S., Boothman, R., Anderson, S., Welch, K., Saint, S., and Rogers, M. (2010, August 17). "Liability Claims and Costs before and after Implementation of a Medical Error Disclosure Program." *Annals of Internal Medicine,* 153(4), 213–221. doi:10.7326/0003-4819-153-4-201008170-00002.

Kaiser, C. (2006, February 1). "Saying 'I'm Sorry' Could Stem the Tide of Malpractice Claims—Increasing Numbers of Hospitals, Insurance Carriers and States adopt Full Disclosure Measures to Acknowledge Medical Errors." *Diagnostic Imaging,* 25. Retrieved from https://link.gale.com/apps/doc/A141590582/HRCA?u=txshrpub100514&sid=HRCA&xid=4ba14f80.

Kass, J. S., and Rose, R. V. (2016). "Medical Malpractice Reform: Historical Approaches, Alternative Models, and Communication and Resolution Programs." *AMA Journal of Ethics, 18*(3), 299–310. doi:10.1001/journalofethics.2017.18.3.pfor6-1603.

Kleisiaris, C. F., Sfakianakis, C., and Papathanasiou, I. V. (n.d.). "Health Care Practices in Ancient Greece: The Hippocratic Ideal." *Journal of Medical Ethics and History of Medicine, 7*(6), 2014.

Kohn, L., Corrigan, J., Donaldson, M., and eds. (2000). *To Err is Human: Building a Safer Health System.* Institute of Medicine Committee on Quality of Health Care In America. Washington, DC: National Academies Press.

Lambert, B. L., Centomani, N. M., Smith, K. M., Helmchen, L. A., Bhaumik, D. K., Jalundhwala, Y. J., and McDonald, T. B. (2016). "The 'Seven Pillars' Response to Patient Safety Incidents: Effects on Medical Liability Processes and Outcomes." *Health Research and Educational Trust, 51*(53), 2491–2515. doi:10.1111/1475-6773.12548.

Larson, D. A. (2016). "Medical Malpractice Arbitration: Not Business as Usual." *Arbitration Law Review, 69*(8), 69–93.

Lazare, A. (2004). *On Apology.* New York, NY: Oxford University Press.

Lazare, A. (2006). "Apology in Medical Practice: An Emerging Clinical Skill." *JAMA—Journal of the American Medical Association, 296*, 1401–1404.

Leape, L. (2012, Spring). "Apology for Errors: Whose Responsbility?" *Frontiers of Health Services Management, 28*(3), 3–12.

LeCraw, F. R., Montanera, D., Jackson, J. P., Keys, J. C., Hetzler, D. C., and Mroz, T. A. (2018, February). "Changes in Liability Claims, Costs and Resolution Times Following Introduction of a Communication-and-Resolution Program in Tennessee." *Jouranal of Patient Safety and Risk Management, 23*(1), 13–18. doi:10.1177/1356262217751808.

Ledema, R., Sorensen, R., Manias, E., Tucket, A., Piper, D., Mallock, N., ... Jorm, C. (2008, December). "Patients' and Family Members' Experiences of Open Disclosure Following Adverse Events." *International Journal for Quality in Health Care, 20*(6), 421–432. doi:doi.org/10.1093/intqhc/mzn043.

LeGros, N., and Pinkall, J. D. (2002, Spring). "The New JCAHO Patient Safety Standards and the Disclosure of Unanticipated Outcomes. Joint Commission on Accreditation of Healthcare Organizations." *Journal of Health Law, 35*(2), 189–210.

Lehman, A. G. (2008, May). "Medical Culture and Error Disclosure." *AMA Journal of Ethics, 10*(5), 282–287. doi:10.1001/virtualmentor.2008.10.5.ccas4-0805.

Lidz, J. W. (1995, October 1). "Medicine as a Metaphor in Plato." *The Journal of Medicine & Philosophy, 20*(5), 527–541. doi:doi.org/10.1093/jmp/20.5.527.

Liebman, C. B. (2011, Summer). "Medical Malpractice Mediation: Benefits gained, Opportunities Lost." *Law & Contemporary Problems, 74*(3), 125–149.

Liebman, C. B., and Hyman, C. S. (2004, July/August). "A Mediation Skills Model to Manage Disclosure of Errors and Adverse Events to Patients." *Health Affairs, 23*(4), 22–32. doi:10.1377/hlthaff.23.4.22.

Liebman, C. B., and Hyman, C. S. (2005). "Medical Error Disclosure, Mediation Skills and Malpractice Litigation." Retrieved from The Pew Charitable Trusts—The Project on Medical Liability in Pennsylvania: https://www.pewtrusts.org/-/media/legacy/uploadedfiles/wwwpewtrustsorg/reports/medical_liability/liebmanreportpdf.pdf.

Makary, M., and Daniel, M. (2016, May 3). "Medical Error—The Third Leading Cause of Death in the U.S." *British Medical Journal*(2139), 353. doi:10.1136/bmj.i2139.

Mapes, C. (1898). "Shall Patients Be Informed that They Have Cancer or Syphilis?" *New York Medical Journal*(5), 560–562.

Marcus, L. (2002). "A Culture of Conflict: Lessons from Rengotiating Healthcare." *Journal of Health Care Law & Policy*, 5, 447–454.

Mastroianni, A., Mello, M., Sommer, S., Hardy, M., and Gallagher, T. (2010, September). "The Flaws in State "Apology" and "Disclosure" Laws Dilute Their Intended Impact on Malpractice Suits." *Health Affairs*, 29(9), 1611–1619. doi:0.1377/hlthaff.2009.0134.

McDonald, T., Helmchen, L., Smith, K., Centomani, N., Gunderson, A., Mayer, D., and Chamberlin, W. (2010). "Responding to Patient Safety Incidents: The 'Seven Pillars.'" *Quality & Safety in Health Care*, 9, 1–4. doi:10.1136/qshc.2008.031633.

McMichael, B. J. (2018, March). "The Failure of 'Sorry': An Empirical Evaluation of Apology Laws, Health Care and Medical Malpractice." *Lewis & Clark Law Review*, 22(4), 1200–1263.

McMichael, B. J., and Van Horn, R. L. (2019, May 14). "How to Apologize Effectively for Medical Errors." Retrieved from Healio Primary Care: https://www.healio.com/primary-care/practice-management/news/online/%7B8ed41e3b-5695-40bd-aaf3-0831ed2bcb4d%7D/how-to-apologize-effectively-for-medical-errors.

McMichael, B. J., Van Horn, R., and Viscusi, W. (2019, February). "'Sorry' Is Never Enough: How State Apology Laws Fail to Reduce Medical Malpractice Liability Risk." *Stanford Law Review, 71*(2), 341.

Mello, M. M., Boothman, R. C., McDonald, T., Driver, J., Lembitz, A., Boumeester, D., ... Gallagher, T. (2014). "Communication-and-Resolution Programs: The Challengs and Lessons Learned from Six Early Adopters." *Health Affairs, 33*(1), 20–29. doi:10.1377/hlthaff.2013.0828.

Mello, M., Armstrong, S., Greenberg, Y., McCotter, P., and Gallagher, T. (2016). "Challenges of Implementing a Communication-and-Resolution Program Where Multiple Organizations Must Cooperate." *Health Services Research, 51*(6), 2550-2568.

Miles, S. H. (2004). *The Hippocratic Oath and the Ethics of Medicine.* New York, NY: Oxford University Press.

Miles, S. H. (2009, October 17). "Hippocrates and Informed Consent." *The Lancet, 374*(9698), P1322–P1323. doi:10.1016/S0140-6736(09)61812-2.

Mills, D. H. (1977). *Report on the Medical Insurance Feasibility Study.* California Medical Association. San Fransisco, CA: Sutter Publications.

Mulholland, B. (2017, July 24). "8 Critical Change Management Models to Evolve and Survive." Retrieved from Process.st: https://www.process.st/change-management-models/.

Neumann, M., Scheffer, C., Tauschel, D., Lutz, G., Wirtz, M., and Edelhauser, F. (2012). "Physcian Empathy: Definition, Outcome-Relevance and Its Measurement in Patient Care and Medical

Education." *GMS Zeitscrhift fure Medizinische Ausbildung, 29*(1). doi:0.3205/zma000781.

NIH Clinical Center. (2019, November 15). *Patient Bill of Rights*. Retrieved from National Institutes of Health Clinical Center: https://clinicalcenter.nih.gov/participate/patientinfo/legal/bill_of_rights.html.

Okimoto, T. G., Wenzel, M., and Hedrick, K. (2013, February). "Refusing to Apologize Can Have Psychologcal Benefits (and We Issue No Mea Culpa for This Research Finding." *European Journal of Social Psychology, 43*(1), 22–31. doi:10.1002/ejsp.1901.

O'Reilly, K. B. (2018, January 26). "1 in 3 Physicians Has Been Sued; By Age 55, 1 in 2 Hit with Suit." Retrieved from American Medical Association: https://www.ama-assn.org/practice-management/sustainability/1-3-physicians-has-been-sued-age-55-1-2-hit-suit.

Palatnik, A. M. (2016, September). "To Err Is Human." *Nursing Critical Care, 11*(5), 4. doi:10.1097/01.CCN.0000490961.44977.8d.

Peskin, S. M. (2018, October 4). "My Human Doctor." Retrieved from *New York Times*: https://www.nytimes.com/2018/10/04/well/live/doctors-errors-apologies.html.

Peter G. .Peterson Foundation. (2019, July 22). "How Does the U.S. Healthcare System Compare to Other Countries?" Retrieved from Peter G. Peterson Foundation: https://www.pgpf.org/blog/2019/07/how-does-the-us-healthcare-system-compare-to-other-countries.

Poorolajal, J., Rezaie, S., and Aghighi, N. (2015, January 1). "Barriers to Medical Error Reporting." *International Journal of Preventative Medicine, 6*(1), 97.

Robbennolt, J. (2003). "Apologies and Legal Settlement: An Empiracl Examination." *Michigan Law Review*, 460–570.

Roberts, R. G. (2997, July-August). "The Art of Apology: When and How to Seek Forgiveness." *FPM—American Academy of Family Physicians, 14*(17), 44–49.

Sage, W. (2005). "Medical Malpractice Insurance and the Emperor's Clothes." *DePaul Law Review, 54*, 463–464.

Sage, W. M. (2004). "The Forgotten Third: Liability Insurance and the Medical Malpractice Crisis." *Health Affairs, 23*, 11–12.

Schoenewolf, G. (2015, February 2). "6 Kinds of Apology and What They Mean." Retrieved from PsychCentral: https://blogs.psychcentral.com/psychoanalysis-now/2015/02/6-kinds-of-apology-and-what-they-mean/.

Shaprio, R., Simpson, D., Lawrence, S., Talsky, A., Sobocinski, K., and Schiedermayer, D. (1989). "A Survey of Sued and Nonsued Physicians and Suing Patients." *Archives of Internal Medicine, 149*(10), 2190–2196.

Shmerling, R. H. (2015, November 25). "The Myth of the Hippocratic Oath." Retrieved from Harvard Health Publishing—Harvard Medical School: https://www.health.harvard.edu/blog/the-myth-of-the-hippocratic-oath-201511258447.

Shorter, E. (1985). *Bedside Manners: The Troubled History of Doctors and Patients*. New York, NY: Simon and Schuster.

Smith, A. (2019, May 9). "Deny, Defend, Death: A Newborn's Death and Salt in the Wound." Retrieved from Physician Leaders: https://www.physicianleaders.org/news/deny-defend-death-salt-wound.

Smith, A. (2019, May 10). "Medical Errors and CRP: Beyond Denial and Defense." Retrieved from American Association for

Physician Leadership: https://www.physicianleaders.org/news/medical-errors-crp-beyond-denial-and-defense.

Sohn, D. H., and Bal, B. S. (2012, May). "Medical Malpractice Reform: The Role of Alternative Dispute Resolution." *Clinical Orthopaedics and Related Researc, 470*(5), 1370–1378. doi:10.1007/s11999-011-2206-2.

Sokol, D. K. (2006, December). "How the Doctor's Nose Has Shortened over Time: A Historical Overview of the Truth-Telling Debate in the Doctor-Patient Relationship." *Journal of the Royal Society of Medicine, 99*(12), 632–636. doi:10.1258/jrsm.99.12.632.

Sorrell, J. (2017, March 7). "Ethics: Ethical Issues with Medical Errors—Shaping a Culture of Safety in Healthcare." *OJIN: Online Journal of Issues in Nursing, 22*(2). Retrieved from http://ojin.nursingworld.org/MainMenuCategories/ANAMarketplace/ANAPeriodicals/OJIN/Columns/Ethics/Ethical-Issues-with-Medical-Errors.html.

*SorryWorks! (Our Approach).* (2019). Retrieved from SorryWorks!: https://sorryworks.net/our-approach.

Spiegel, A. D. (1997, May 1). "Hammurabi's Managed Health Care—Circa 1700 B.C." Retrieved from Managed Care: https://www.managedcaremag.com/archives/1997/5/hammurabis-managed-health-care-circa-1700-bc.

Stanford Encyclopedia of Philosophy. (2014, August 3). "Ancient Ethical Theory." Retrieved from Stanford Encyclopedia of Philosophy: https://plato.stanford.edu/entries/ethics-ancient/#2.

Staszak, S. (2019, April). "In the Shadow of Litigation: Arbitration and Medical Malpractice Reform." *Journal of Health Politics, Policy and Law, 44*(2), 267–301. doi:doi.org/10.1215/03616878-7277380.

Studdert, D., Mello, M., Gawande, A., Brennan, T., and Wang, Y. (2007, January). "Disclosure of Medical Injury to Patients: An Improbable Risk Management Strategy." *Health Affairs, 26*(1), 215–226. doi:10.1377/hlthaff.26.1.215.

Studdert, D., Mello, M., and Brennan, T. (2004). "Health Policy Report: Medical Malpractice." *New England Journal of Medicine, 350*(6), 283–292.

Supra, J.D. (2019, September 18). "5 Ways Mediators Can Add Value to Hospital Communication and Resolution Programs." Retrieved from JDSupra.com: https://www.jdsupra.com/legalnews/how-mediators-can-add-value-to-hospital-32396/.

Taft, L. (2005, Winter). "Apology and Medical Mistake: Opportunity or Foil?" *Annals of Health Law, 14*(1), 55–94.

Tan, S. (2015, January 27). "Patient Safety and Tort Reform." Retrieved from Clinical and Neurology News: https://www.mdedge.com/clinicalneurologynews/article/96700/patient-safety-and-tort-reform.

Tan, Z. Y. (2016, August 22). "Hospitals Rethink "Deny-and-Defend" Approach to Medical Error." Retrieved from Medical City News: https://medcitynews.com/2016/08/hospitals-rethink-medical-error/.

Tavuchis, N. (1991). *Mea Culpa: A Sociology of Apology and Reconciliation.* Stanford, CA: Stanford University Press.

Wallace, R. A. (2017, September-October). "A Brief History of Medical Liability Litigation and Insurance." *West Virginia Medicial Journal, 113,* 6–9.

Waxman, O. B. (2017, July 15). "How the Public Learned about the Infamous Tuskegee Syphilis Study." Retrieved from *Time* magazine: https://time.com/4867267/tuskegee-syphilis-study/.

Welch, S. J. (2011, March). "Quality Matters: Deny and Defend—Apologizing Hampered by Physician Culture, Risk Management." *Emergency Medicine News, 33*(3), 12–24. doi:10.1097/01.EEM.0000395426.55635.4c.

Winch, G. (2010, December 9). "The Science of Effective Apologies." doi:https://www.psychologytoday.com/us/blog/the-squeaky-wheel/201012/the-science-effective-apologies.

Wojcieszak, D., Banja, J., and Houk, C. (2006, June). "The Sorry Works! Coalition: Making the Case for Full Disclosure." *Journal on Quality and Patient Safety, 32*(6), 344–350.

Worthington, E., and Scherer, M. (2004). "Forgiveness Is an Emotional-Focussed Coping Strategy That Can Reduce Health Risks and Promote Health Resilience: Theory, Review and Hypothesis." *Psychological Health, 19,* 385–405.

Wu, A. (2000, March). "Medical Error: The Second Victim." *British Medical Journal, 320,* 726. doi:10.1136/bmj.320.7237.726.

Wu, A., Cavanaugh, T., McPhee, S., Lo, B., and Micco, G. (1997). "To Tell the Truth: Ethical and Practical Issues in Disclosing Medical Mistakes to Patients." *Journal of General Internal Medicine, 12*(12), 770–775.

Zimmerman, T., and Amori, G. (2007). "Including Patients in Root Cause and System and Failure Analysis: Legal and Psychological Implications." *Journal of Healthcare Risk Management, 27,* 27–34.

# INDEX

## A

abandonment, feelings of by patient, 63–64
Ackerman, B. G., 62, 65
active listening, use of, 116, 131
adverse event, defined, 5
adverse medical event, use of term, 7
Agency for Healthcare Research and Quality, "Communication and Optimal Resolution Toolkit" (CANDOR), 132–134
Allan, A., 74–75, 127
alternative dispute resolution (ADR)
  apology programs and CRPs as compared to, 131
  defined, 112–114
  in light of medical error, 125
  role of, 110, 111
  and success rate in avoiding litigation, 113
Alzheimer's Association, report on patients' knowledge of their diagnosis, 20
*American College of Physicians Ethics Manual*, 89

American Hospital Association (AHA), "A Patient's Bill of Rights," 19
American Medical Association (AMA)
  Code of Ethics, 15
  Code of Ethics of, 14
  Council on Ethical and Judicial Affairs, 89
  report on medical liability lawsuits, 97, 99
American Society for Health Care Risk Management, on ERM system's guiding principles, 174–175
anesthesia, and medical malpractice litigation, 26
anger, feelings of by patient, 64, 94
anxiety, physicians and health-care providers as suffering from when it comes to restrictions and concerns about what they are and are not allowed to discuss, 168
"Apology" (Socrates), 31
apology laws, 24, 88–96, 151, 163–164
apology training programs
  recommendation for, 68, 182
  resistance to, 68–69

apology/apologizing
  in ADR techniques, 112–113
  anatomy of, 71–96
  art of, 77–79
  basic ingredients of, 72
  benefits of, 73–77
  consequences of, 70, 126, 127
  defined, 71–72
  difficulties in physicians' use of, 7
  lack of effective system for, 60–61
  lack of in medicine, 54–61
  lack of sufficient skills in making of, 59–60
  and litigation, 155–179
  need for, xx
  positive physical ramifications of, 74
  problems with, 7
  and reduction in frequency and size of medical malpractice claims, 172
  reluctance to, 84–88
  risk managers and, 57–58
  sorry as working, to an extent, 170–173
  steps of effective apology, 159–165
  steps toward proper apology, according to Maimonides, 78–79
  from systems versus from individuals, 58–59
  as therapeutic, 72–73
  training in, 166–168. *See also* apology training programs
  types of, 79–84
  well-crafted one as key to forgiveness, 75
  "worst apology," 78
arbitration, use of, 112, 114, 121–125, 131
Aristotle, 32–33

Asclepieion medical practice, school of, 12
Associated Press, on Tuskegee study, 19
autonomy, principle of, 30, 40, 42, 115

**B**

Babylonia, and history of medicine, 11
bad news, practitioners as underestimating patients' abilities to accept, 18
Barbe, David O., 99
beneficence, principle of, 30, 39–40, 53
Berdine, G., 35, 36
betrayal, feelings of patient by, 64, 94
bill of rights (for patient), 19, 38–41
Blackstone, William, 26
Bohnen, J. M., 3
Boothman, Rick, 46, 49, 54–55, 105, 128–129, 136, 138, 139, 140
Brennan, T. A., 55
*British Medical Journal*, study on medical error, 6–7

**C**

CANDOR ("Communication and Optimal Resolution Toolkit"), 132–134, 150
Carroll, A. E., 101
Cathell, D. W., 14
Chamberlain, C. J., 4, 154
China, yin and yang balances as focus in, 11
clinical/patient safety risks, 175, 176–178
Clinton, Hillary, 24
closure, impact of apology on, 70
Code of Hammurabi/Hammurabi Code, 10–11, 12, 25–26, 67

collaborative-communication-and-resolution program (CCRP), 130
commission, errors of, 2, 3, 8
Committee on Quality Health Care in America (IOM), 21–22
"Communication and Optimal Resolution Toolkit" (CANDOR), 132–134, 150
communication-and-resolution program (CRP)
   effectiveness and rollout of, 150–152
   funding for from Daley Ullem settlement, xvi
   use of, 126–134
complication, defined, 5
COPIC Insurance Co., as disclosure/CRP case study, 143–144, 146, 150
Cos school, 13
Council on Ethical and Judicial Affairs (AMA), 89
cover-ups, use of, 49

# D

Daley Ullem, Beth, xv–xviii, xix, 28, 58, 86, 87, 107, 157, 175–176, 177
Damianakis, T., 5
Daniel, M., 6, 7
deception, use of, 14–15
deny-and-defend culture
   benefits in erosion of, 171
   concept behind, 43
   downfalls from, 44–45, 168
   elements of, 46
   factors blamed for, 48–54
   fall back to, 106
   negative outcomes of, 47
   as not way to prevent litigation, 8
   responses in as compared to CANDOR responses, 133–134
   start of in ancient Mesopotamia, 11
   use of term, xix
disclosure
   all disclosure, all the time, 153–154
   case studies in, 135–144
   discomfort with as factor in deny-and-defend mind-set, 51–52
   effectiveness and rollout of programs of, 150–152
   Hippocrates's foggy approach to error disclosure, 34–38
   malpractice litigation as wrong way to encourage, 28
   in modern ethical models, 38
   as not always forthcoming, 29
   physicians as moving away from, 14–15
   physicians as slowly leaning toward more disclosure, 69
   process of, 152–153
   reason for doctors not disclosing, 17
   successes and challenges through programs of, 145–149
   3R program of, 143–144
   variation in, 69
"do no harm," 29, 34, 35, 36, 42, 153
doctor-patient relationship. *See* physician-patient relationship
doctors. *See* physicians

# E

Eastern medicine, 11
eclectics, as competitors to physicians, 16
Egypt, and history of medicine, 11
empathy, 165–166
enterprise risk management (ERM), implementation of, 173–179
Etchegaray, J. M., 170

## F

flight-or-fight reflexes, as factor in deny-and-defend mind-set, 49–50
Florida, apology law in, 89
forgiveness
  as aspect of apology, 72, 168
  benefits of, 74, 76–77
  generating of, 155–156
  during Judaism's Days of Awe, 79
  paving way toward, 126, 127
  well-crafted apology as key to, 75
Friedman, Heshy, 78
full apology laws, 92–93

## G

Gallagher, T. H., 69, 164
Gillies, R. A., 166–167
Gisborne, Thomas, 17–18
Golann, D., 104, 106
Gorski, D., 7
government, role of in safety of citizens, 18–19
Greece (ancient)
  attitudes of toward medical ethics, 30–38
  and history of medicine, 11–13
  pledges to pagan deities in, 34
Gregory, John, 14–15
Grober, E. D., 3
guilt, feelings of when mistakes are made, 56, 66

## H

Hammurabi, 10–11, 25–26, 43, 67
harm, "do no harm," 29, 34, 35, 36, 42, 153
health-care industry
  deny-and-defend culture of, xix, 11, 42–48. *See also* deny-and-defend culture
  fingerpointing culture in, 48
  physicians' progressive movement in, 20
Helo, S., 65, 66, 68
Hilfiker, David, 126–127, 171
Hippocrates, 12–13, 34–38
Hippocratic Oath, 13, 30, 34, 36–37
homeopaths, as competitors to physicians, 16
honesty
  beneficence as mandating, 39
  benefits of, 50
  as best policy, 41, 75
  as core of UMHS, 138
  in early adaptors of CRP model, 146
  impact of lack of, 74
  importance of in Cos school, 13
  as more of a given, 20
  in philosophies of ancient ethicists, 30, 31, 33
*The Honeymooners* (TV show), "worst apology" on, 78
Hyman, Chris Stern, 116–117, 119, 120

## I

India, Vedic medicine in, 11
Institute of Medicine (IOM), *To Err Is Human: Building a Safer Health System*, 5, 21–25, 27–28

## J

Johnson, Lyndon B., 18
Joint Commission on the Accreditation of Hospital Organizations, 24, 89
Judaism, on art of apologizing, 77–78, 79
justice, principle of, 40–41

## K

Kaiser Permanente, and arbitrated disputes, 122, 123

## L

Lambert, B. L., 142
Larson, D. A., 123, 124
law
  link of medicine to, 25–28
  malpractice industry and advice of legal counsel as factor in deny-and-defend mind-set, 50–51
lawsuits/litigation. *See also* malpractice lawsuit/litigation
  apologizing and, 155–179
  as current reaction to adverse medical events, 25
  by Daley Ullem, xvi–xviii, 28, 107
  impact of apology on, 70
  reasons for, 47, 64
  time and expenses in, 45, 55, 122, 124, 128
Lazare, A., 72
Leape, L. L., 59, 68, 76, 157, 158, 159
Lehman, A. G., 53, 61
Lidz, J. W., 32
Liebman, Carole, 116–117, 119–120
lying, admitting of by physicians, 18

## M

Maimonides, 78–79
Makary, M., 6, 7
malpractice
  as cost of doing business, 97
  first case of in America, 26
  legal remedies for, 26
malpractice industry, as factor in deny-and-defend mind-set, 50–51
malpractice insurance, 45, 50, 124, 141

malpractice lawsuit/litigation
  as current reaction to adverse medical events, 25
  dropping of cases in, 104–105
  failure of, 97–110
  physicians' view of, 55
  role of trial lawyers in handling of, 102–103, 106
  as worst tool for dealing with medical mistakes or encouraging disclosure of such mistakes, 108–109
managed medical care, 11
McCoy, Michael, 99–100
McDonald, T., 143
McKillop, D., 74–75, 127
McMichael, Benjamin, 90–91, 94, 95–96, 173
Mediating Suits against Hospitals (MeSH), 118
mediation, use of, 112, 114–121, 131, 132
Medicaid, 18
medical errors
  according to Grober and Bohnen, 3
  as active or passive, 3
  ADR in light of, 125
  awareness of, xviii–xix
  as breach of physician's duties, 5
  defining of, 1–6
  examples of, 3, 4, 5
  lack of effective reporting system for, 60–61
  metrics of, 6–7, 25
  as outlined in *To Err Is Human*, 21–22
  silence as worst way to deal with, 182
  use of term, 7
  what patients need/want regarding, 156–159

medical ethics
  according to ancient philosophers, 30–38
  modern models of, 38–41
medical malpractice, legal remedies for, 26
medical mistakes, use of term, 7
medical schools
  and ethical quandaries, 59
  history of, 15–16
  training in apologizing, 166–167. See also apology training programs
Medicare, 18
medicine
  culture of as tending to lead to focus on deny-and-defend, 53
  as dangerous profession, xvii, 65, 105, 183
  history of, 9–13
  inherent risks in, 114
  link of to law, 25–28
Mello, M. M., 55, 149, 150–151
mercury, use of in medicine, 16
MeSH (Mediating Suits against Hospitals), 118
Mesopotamia, and Hammurabi Code, 10–11
Miles, S. H., 37
mistakes
  discomfort in acknowledgment of, 56–57
  as fact of life in most industries, 54
  malpractice lawsuit/litigation as worst tool for dealing with medical mistakes, 108–109
  no room for in modern medicine, according to Wu, 67–68
  physicians as feeling guilt and shame from making of, 56, 66
  physicians as not having outlet for guilt and shame that comes with making of, 68
  use of term "medical mistakes," 7
"Morbidity and Mortality" conferences, 60
Moulton, C.-A. E., 65, 66, 68

# N

National Institutes of Health Clinical Center, bill of rights, 38–39
National Medical Error Disclosure and Compensation Act (MEDiC), 24, 88
National Practitioner Data Bank (NPDB), 148
Nevada, apology law in, 89
*New England Journal of Medicine*, on National Medical Error Disclosure and Compensation Act (MEDiC), 24
New York City Health and Hospitals Corp (HHC), examination of cases brought against, 118
nonmaleficence, principle of, 29, 30, 35, 39, 53
"not sorry"
  impact of on patients, 62–64
  impact of on physicians, 65–70
*Nursing Critical Care*, Palatnik guest editorial in, 25

# O

Obama, Barack, 24
O'Brien, Sharon, 171–172
Okimoto, T. G., 71–72, 85, 86
omission, errors of, 2, 3, 8, 40
operational risks, 175–176

## P

Palatnik, Anne Marie, 25
partial apology laws, 92
patient distress, as factor in deny-and-defend mind-set, 52
patients
   feelings of abandonment, anger, and betrayal by, 63–64, 94
   impact of "not sorry" on, 62–64
   involvement of in apologizing, 168–170
   practitioners as underestimating patients' abilities to accept bad news, 18
   what wronged patients need, 156–159
patient's bill of rights, 19, 38–41
Pennsylvania, apology law in, 89
Percival, Thomas, 14–15
Peskin, Sara, 60, 61
Pew Demonstration Mediation and ADR Project, 117, 120
Pho, L., 5
physician-patient relationship, 13–15, 19, 29, 30, 59, 64, 137, 154, 171
physicians
   admitting to lying by, 18
   competitors to, 16
   feelings of guilt when mistakes are made by, 56, 66
   impact of "not sorry" on, 65–70
   as not having outlet for guilt and shame that comes with making mistakes, 68
   personal duties of, 29–30
   progressive movement of in health-care industry, 20
   as "second victims" in adverse medical events, 66–67, 76, 127
   view of malpractice lawsuit/litigation by, 55
Plato, 31–32
pretrial screenings, use of, 112, 113, 114
preventative medicine, origin of concept of, 12
public. *See also* patients
   and apologizing on demand, 80–81
   pressure by, 162
   relationship of with health-care practitioners, 19

## R

risk management/risk managers
   and apologies, 57–58
   enterprise risk management (ERM), 173–179
   in health-care system, 43–44, 46, 51, 55–56, 57–58, 62, 98, 101, 136, 143, 183
Roman law (ancient), and medical malpractice, 26

## S

Sage, W., 55
Schoenewolf, G., 79–84
Scott (author), 66
"second victims," physicians as in adverse medical event, 66–67, 76, 127
secrecy, cult of/culture of, 13–20, 28, 35, 43–54, 94
"Seven Pillars" strategy, 130, 140–141, 142, 143
shame, feelings of when mistakes are made, 56, 66
silence
   according to Hippocrates, 38
   breaking the wall of, 114, 131
   cautions for, 44

consequences of, 64, 70, 75, 98, 100, 101–102
as conspiracy, xvi, xvii, xviii, 52
culture of, 17, 68
reasons for, xix, 55, 60–61, 131
as worst way to deal with medical error, 182
Sisk (author), 13–14
"snake oil" salesmen, as competitors to physicians, 16
Social Security, expansion of to include Medicare and Medicaid, 18
Socrates, 31
Sokol, D. K., 13, 29
Sorry Works! Coalition, 170
Spiegel, A. D., 11
Stanford University Medical Indemnity and Trust Insurance Company, 146
Staszak, S., 122–123, 124
stonewalling, use of, xv, 44, 47, 64, 98, 107, 108, 112, 177
Studdert, D., 55
system failure, as factor in deny-and-defend mind-set, 48–49

# T

Tavuchis, Nicholas, 161
*teshuva*, concept of, 79
3R program of disclosure, 143–144
*To Err Is Human: Building a Safer Health System* (Institute of Medicine report), 5–6, 21–25, 27–28
tort reform, apology laws as part of, 89, 91
Tourangeau, A., 5
transparency
  apology/disclosure as providing, 84, 127, 135

benefits of, 131, 143, 145
Boothman's idea for, 129
call for, 19–20
consequences of lack of, 44
as essential to success of disclosure programs, 149
increase in, 25
in UMHS approach, 88, 135–136, 138
Tuskegee study, 19

# U

University of Illinois Chicago Medical Center (UMCC)
  as disclosure/CRP case study, 140–143, 146, 150
  study on implementation of "Seven Pillars" strategy, 130
University of Michigan Health System (UMHS), as disclosure/CRP case study, 54, 135–140, 146, 150, 172–173

# V

Vedic medicine, 11

# W

Wagner, L. M., 5
Waite (author), 145–146
*Washington Post*, Ackerman's discussion of emotional reactions to medical errors in, 62
West Virginia Mutual Insurance Company and Conveys (formerly ProMutual Group), 146
Western medicine, birth of, 12
Winch, G., 72
wrongdoing

admitting of, xvii, xix–xx, 16, 43, 77, 84–85, 86, 90, 167, 171, 178
difficulty in acknowledgment of, 8, 28, 51–52, 54, 55, 56, 84, 88
impact of forcing physicians to apologize for, 91
medical establishment's attempt to repudiate culpability for, 43

patients as expecting acknowledgment of, 156
refusal to admit, 109
wronged patients, what they need, 156–159
Wu, Albert, 64, 66–68, 127

## Y

yin and yang balances, 11

www.ingramcontent.com/pod-product-compliance
Lightning Source LLC
Chambersburg PA
CBHW031839170526
45157CB00001B/355